FISMAN'S FRAUD: THE ACCOMPLICES

Supplementary Reference

A collection of letters and correspondences

By R.N. Watteel, PhD Statistics

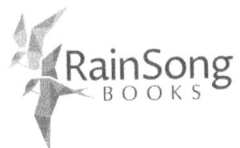

An Imprint of Whisperwood Publishing | Canada

Copyright © 2023 R.N. Watteel, PhD Statistics

All rights reserved.

ISBN: 978-1-988363-26-4 (paperback)

This is a work of nonfiction. No names have been changed, no characters invented, no events fabricated. I am not a lawyer; views do not represent legal opinion. I have made every effort to ensure that the information in this book was correct at press time. Views are my own based on evidence as referenced in the book. Readers are encouraged to assess the evidence presented in order to draw their own conclusions.

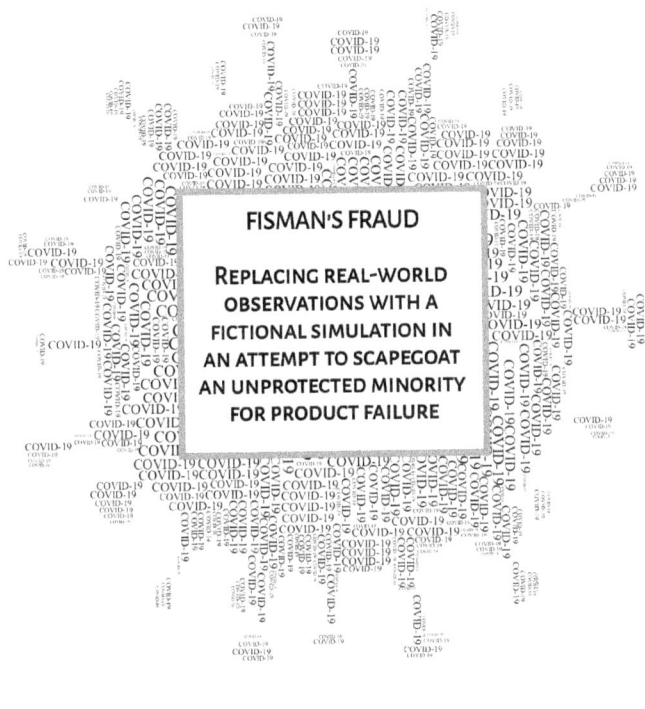

This supplementary reference guide provides a collection of letters, documents and correspondences between R.N. Watteel and the Canadian Medical Association Journal (CMAJ), the University of Toronto (U of T) and the Canadian Institutes of Health Research (CIHR) regarding the research study coauthored by David Fisman, Afia Amoako and Ashleigh Tuite entitled: *Impact of population mixing between vaccinated and unvaccinated subpopulations on infectious disease dynamics: implications for SARS-CoV-2 transmission;* CMAJ 2022;194:E573-E580.

CONTENTS

Introduction 1
    Background 1
    Contents 5
    Evidentiary Timeline 6
CMAJ Letters 8
    e-Letter Submitted through the CMAJ Portal 9
    Letter Couriered to CMAJ 11
    Email Correspondence 12
Letters to the University of Toronto 14
    First Letter to University of Toronto & Response 15
    Second Letter to University of Toronto & Response 18
    Third Letter to U of T, cc'd: CIHR, CMAJ 21
University of Toronto Final Response & Decision 26
Letters to CIHR 27
    Letter to CIHR: Misconduct Allegations 28
    Letter to CIHR: Breach of Policy by UofT 29
    Email Correspondence with CIHR 34
Letter to Ontario Premier Ford 43
Appendix A: Critique of CMAJ Study 46
    Summary 46
    Concern #1: Overt Bias 48

Concern #2: Poorly constructed, inadequate modelling ... 49

Concern #3: Failure to capture real-world trends ... 54

Concern #4: Misinterpretation of Results & Societal Harm ... 58

Concern #5: The danger of conflating reality with fiction ... 61

Concern #6: The rampant spread of disinformation ... 64

Concern #7: Blatant scientific and research misconduct ... 68

Bottom Line: RETRACTION and INVESTIGATION are in order ... 72

Notes ... 75

References ... 79

About the Author ... 84

CHAPTER 1

Introduction

The less time you spend with Truth, the easier it is to believe lies.
— LeCrae, Rapper & Songwriter (1979-)

This supplementary guide provides letters and emails referenced in the book entitled *Fisman's Fraud: The Rise of Canadian Hate Science*. It documents efforts to have a heavily cited and far-reaching fraudulent publication retracted, the misconduct investigated and the public record set straight. The study in question, *Impact of population mixing between vaccinated and unvaccinated subpopulations on infectious disease dynamics: implications for SARS-CoV-2 transmission*, was written by University of Toronto researchers and received considerable institutional backing. My correspondences with the affiliated institutions are provided in the chapters that follow.

Background

In late 2021 and into the early months of 2022, with over 80% of the population fully vaccinated with the new genetic COVID-19 vaccines, provinces across Canada witnessed a massive upswing in the number of COVID-19 cases. In an apparent attempt to quell doubt about the effectiveness of the experimental COVID-19 vaccines and to encourage further uptake of the pharmaceuticals, three University of Toronto researchers, David Fisman, Afia Amoako and Ashleigh Tuite, concocted a faux modelling study that sought to scapegoat the "unvaccinated" for the record-breaking surge.

Despite the study's utter detachment from reality and its complete lack of scientific merit, it was published in the peer-reviewed Canadian Medical Association Journal (CMAJ) and backed by both the University of Toronto (U of T) and the Canadian Institutes of Health Research (CIHR). Not only was the research by the trio of unimaginably poor quality, but the researchers attempted to pass off their fictional findings as "fact" (which constitutes scientific fraud) and used their contrivance to advocate for harsh, discriminatory public policy.

The three researchers were highly credentialed in the area of infectious disease epidemiology and mathematical modelling. Yet, irrefutably, statements written in their CMAJ publication purporting to be fact were fabricated and blatantly false. Not only have the researchers held to these false claims under intense criticism from the scientific community, the main author, David Fisman, has continued to promote the harmful falsities and the three institutions have continued to support the fraudulent research.

Simple, routine validity checks show that the models produced by the study did not fit real-world observations; in fact, the results generated *completely contradicted reality.* The lack of model validation wasn't the only glaring omission in the study. No hypothesis was tested and no real-world observations were used. Yet, the research trio drew strong conclusions about the real world.

It is impossible to overstate just how bad the modelling was (an overview is provided in Appendix A). It's no wonder numerous scientists were compelled to publicly critique the study's flaws. Ironically, with so many serious deficiencies demanding attention, it has been easy for critics to get lost in the weeds and overlook the most fundamental issue with the publication:

The authors attempted to pass off their fabricated faux findings, opposite reality, as fact and a true reflection of the real world. That is considered an overt act of scientific fraud.

Fabrication – making up research results and data, and reporting them as a true reflection of events – is, by its very nature, intentional. One simply cannot make up results and report them as facts unknowingly. Their fictitious findings were cited in Parliament and used to justify vaccine mandates and restrictions against those who chose not to take the injections. They claimed such actions were for the greater good.

In the days and weeks following the CMAJ publication, over a hundred national and international news articles cited the findings and warned about the dangers of mixing with the unvaccinated. The false narrative bolstered by the paper continues to be cited as justification for the harsh treatment of the unvaccinated and the punitive restrictions that were imposed against them.

The scope of the fraudulent activity undertaken by the researchers is unprecedented in Canada, extending beyond common schemes into "hate science" – the fabrication or falsification of scientific findings for the purpose of scapegoating an identifiable group. Moreover, there is clear indication that failure to address this misconduct will result in future uptake of this type of activity.

Given the seriousness of the misconduct, I personally reached out to each of the institutions responsible for the oversight of research integrity to seek remedial action. Figure 1 shows the progression of this eighteen-month journey.

As illustrated in Figure 1 and demonstrated by the evidentiary timeline provided at the end of this chapter, I have gone out of my way to extend every professional courtesy to the individuals and institutions involved to resolve this important matter. Unfortunately, my efforts were futile. My searches, however, revealed a deeper network of support for the misconduct and academic malfeasance. The conflicts of interest of the parties involved, the Establishment's willingness to back the knowingly fraudulent research and the societal implications are discussed in *Fisman's Fraud: The Rise of Canadian Hate Science*.

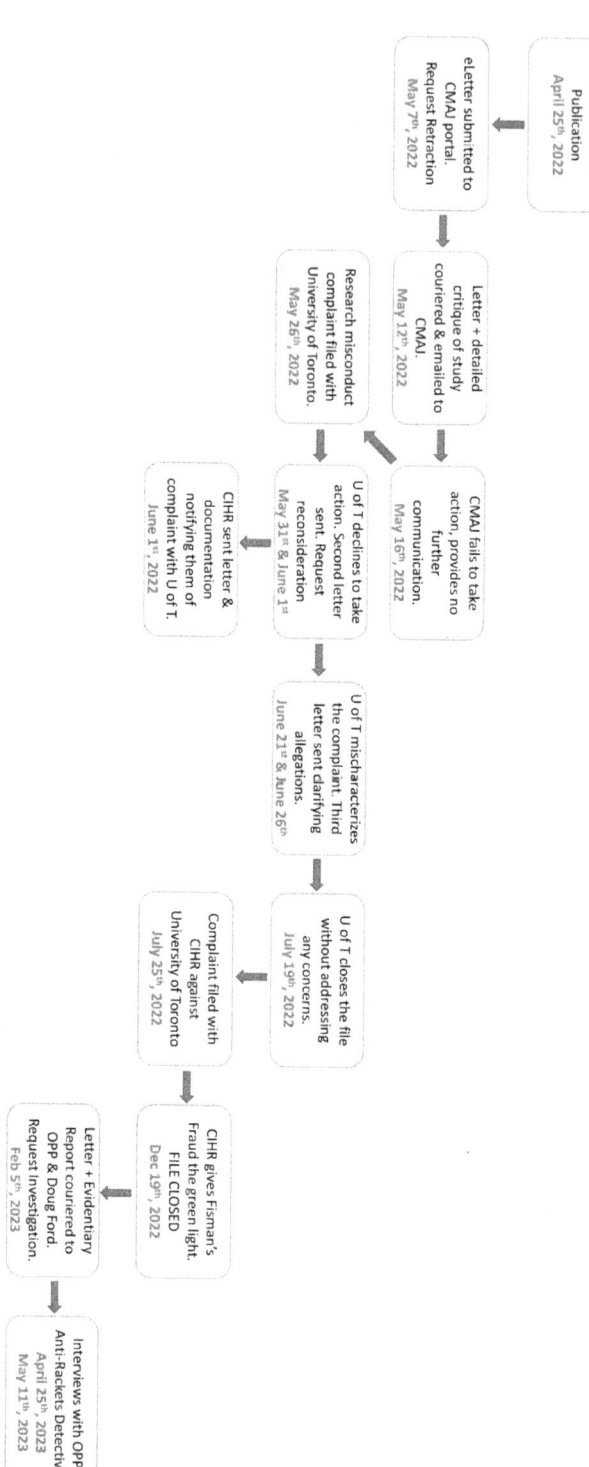

Figure 1: Flowchart of Complaint Progression Against Fisman, Tuite and Amoako

Contents

For transparency, the following documentation is provided in this reference guide:

- ✓ Letters and materials couriered, emailed or directly submitted through the online portal to CMAJ seeking a retraction of the fraudulent study;

- ✓ All letters that were couriered or emailed to the University of Toronto seeking an investigation into the alleged fraud, along with responses received by the university;

- ✓ All correspondence with CIHR regarding the University of Toronto's handling of the scientific fraud allegations and requesting that Parliament be notified of the fraudulent study;

- ✓ The supplementary document that was provided to all three organizations which details the study's complete lack of scientific merit and research integrity (Appendix A). This material establishes the exceptionally low quality of the published research, the researchers' overt prejudice against the individuals they sought to defame and defraud, and it helps establish intent. This material along with the formal letters of complaint demonstrate that the researchers and the affiliated institutions were made fully aware of the fraudulent statements, yet refused to take corrective action.

Additionally, in February 2023, I called on the Anti-Rackets Branch of the Ontario Provincial Police (OPP) to launch a serious police investigation to uncover the true extent of the fraudulent activity, the political involvement and any related racketeering activities or efforts that may have been levied against the Canadian public. Letters requesting an OPP investigation were couriered to Premier Doug Ford and OPP Commissioner Thomas W. B. Carrique along with supporting documentation. The letter provided to Doug Ford is included in the last chapter. The context of the inquiry, my interaction with the OPP and its implications are discussed in *Fisman's Fraud: The Rise of Canadian Hate Science.*

Evidentiary Timeline

Fraudulent study published by CMAJ .... April 25, 2022
Defamatory media blitz commences .... April 25, 2022

e-Letter submitted to CMAJ Portal calling for retraction ...... May 07, 2022
Letter & supporting document couriered to CMAJ .... May 12, 2022
   Delivery verification .... May 16, 2022
email to Kirsten Patrick & CMAJ Editorial Team .... May 16, 2022
   email from CMAJ Group acknowledging receipt .... May 16, 2022
response to CMAJ Group re. online portal submission .... May 16, 2022

Letter & report couriered to UofT: Research Misconduct ...... May 26, 2022
   Delivery verification .... May 30, 2022
eLetter & report to U of T: Research Misconduct .... May 26, 2022
First Response from U of T: Complaint is non-actionable ..... May 31, 2022
Second Letter emailed to U of T: Reconsideration .... June 01, 2022
Second Letter couriered to U of T .... June 07, 2022
   Delivery verification .... June 13, 2022

eLetter & report to CIHR appraising them of situation .... June 01, 2022
Letter & report couriered to CIHR .... June 07, 2022
   Delivery verification .... June 08, 2022

Second Response from UofT: Complaint will not be pursued June 21, 2022
Third Letter couriered to UofT, cc'd: CIHR .... June 26, 2022
   Delivery verification (CIHR) .... June 28, 2022
   Delivery verification (UofT) .... June 28, 2022
Third Letter emailed to UofT, cc'd: CMAJ, CIHR .... June 27, 2022

Third and Final Response from UofT: Case Closed! .... July 19, 2022

eLetter & report to CIHR: Complaint against UoT .... July 25, 2022
Letter & report couriered to CIHR .... July 26, 2022
   Delivery verification (CIHR).. July 27, 2022
First Response from CIHR: Permission to send material...... Aug 18, 2022
First Response to CIHR: Permission granted .... Aug 19, 2022
   Status update requested (no response)........................... Sept 22, 2022
   Status update requested (no response) .... Oct 11, 2022
   Status update requested .... Oct 24, 2022
   Status update received: Decision expected by Nov............ Oct 24, 2022
   Status update requested .... Dec 05, 2022
   Status update received from CIHR: Decision forthcoming.. Dec 09, 2022
CIHR Final Decision: No breach. FILE CLOSED .... Dec 19, 2022

Letter & Report sent to OPP: Request Investigation............. Feb 05, 2023
Interview with OPP Anti-Rackets Detective Sergeant...   Apr 25, 2023
Follow-up call: OPP will not pursue matter .... May 11, 2023

Letter & Report couriered to Doug Ford .... Feb 05, 2023
   No response ....…..   Nov, 2023

Book — Fisman's Fraud: The Rise of Canadian Hate Science.. Nov, 2023

* Many of the letters written to the institutions were delivered by both courier and email. In such cases, the emailed copies are not included in this reference guide in order to reduce duplication.

Chapter 2

CMAJ Letters

"Let's be clear: the work of science has nothing whatever to do with consensus. Consensus is the business of politics. Science, on the contrary, requires only one investigator who happens to be right, which means that he or she has results that are verifiable by reference to the real world."
— Michael Crichton (2003), Writer & Filmmaker

Apart from a form letter and an auto-generated acknowledgment of receipt of materials, CMAJ did not respond to my letters or address the concerns raised. At the time of the paper's submission, Kirsten Patrick was serving as CMAJ's interim editor-in-chief. University of Toronto Professor Andreas Laupacis, the former editor in chief, was serving as senior deputy editor of CMAJ.

In addition to the letters and emails presented in this chapter, CMAJ was copied on the third letter to the University of Toronto that is included in the next chapter and provided with the supplementary material in Appendix A. They had also received an earlier version of the supplementary document on May 11, 2022. Only the second version that was provided to all three institutes is included in the appendix to avoid duplication.

e-Letter Submitted through the CMAJ Portal

e-Letter to CMAJ Submitted May 7th 2022 by Regina N. Watteel

Title: The Fisman et al. SARS-Cov-2 population mixing study FLIPS reality to inform policy and punish the unvaccinated.

A simple deterministic model was developed to simulate hypothetical outcomes of incident cases in Ontario under various group mixing scenarios. The model itself is wholly inadequate, poorly constructed, the baseline conditions are vaguely specified, key parameters and classifications poorly defined, model assumptions highly biased and the interpretation of their results fundamentally flawed.

Perhaps the most important shortcoming of this modelling exercise is that it lacks any meaningful hypothesis or model fitting. To be clear:

(1) No hypothesis is being tested and no observational data is modelled in this study, therefore no meaningful inferences can be drawn about the real-world impact of population mixing regarding SARS-CoV-2 transmission;

(2) This is not a factual study. The model is exploratory in nature with absolutely no benchmarking or validation of any kind.

Moreover, their results follow from basic diffusion principles. The authors concocted a model that simply projects their false expectations. Nothing more. The conclusion "we found that the choices made by people who forgo vaccination contribute disproportionately to risk among those who do get vaccinated" is clearly erroneous given that no people were involved in this study. No real-world observations were used at all.

The authors make no attempt to test their model or to reconcile the obvious discrepancy between the incidence rates produced by their model and the actual incidence rates observed during the Dec. 2021 – Jan. 2022 epidemic wave, the first true test of the vaccination strategy in Canada. Incredulously, the authors then proceed to use the simulated outcomes from their modelling exercise as a basis to inform public policy whilst failing to even recognize the necessity of looking at the actual real-world outcomes! A quick visit to the official Ontario Covid-19 website [2] uncovers a stark contrast between reality and the authors' "findings." Indeed, the simulated results are opposite to the reality that played out in Ontario during the Dec/Jan epidemic wave.

In short, the study concocted a model simulation that FLIPPED reality, then proceeded to inform policy based on it. More specifically, the study leveraged a false premise to support public policy aimed at enhancing vaccine uptake and limiting access to public spaces for unvaccinated people.

This critically flawed work is highly divisive. The quick dissemination of the fictitious findings has resulted in the propagation of fear, mistrust, and derisive attitudes towards a segment of the population in the real world who bear absolutely no resemblance to the entities in Fisman et al.'s model.

We cannot pretend that the epidemic wave in Dec/Jan never happened and simply overwrite it with a faulty simulation that says the opposite. I request that CMAJ retract this paper.

---

* The following automated response was generated by CMAJ upon submission:

> "Thank you for your response. We intend to publish as rapidly as possible all responses that contribute substantially to the topic under discussion."

** CMAJ chose not to publish my eLetter response to the faux study.

Letter Couriered to CMAJ

May 12th, 2022
Kirsten Patrick, Editor-in-Chief
Canadian Medical Association Journal
1410 Blair Towers Place, Suite 500
Ottawa ON, K1J 9B9

Request for Retraction & Investigation into Scientific Misconduct: CMAJ 2022;194:E573-E580

Dear Kirsten Patrick and the CMAJ Editorial Team:

I have serious concerns regarding the scientific quality, integrity and ethics of the Fisman et al. study published by CMAJ on April 25th, 2022:

> David N. Fisman, Afia Amoako, Ashleigh R. Tuite. Impact of population mixing between vaccinated and unvaccinated subpopulations on infectious disease dynamics: implications for SARS-CoV-2 transmission. CMAJ 2022;194:E573-E580

I have put together a comprehensive critique of the paper, discussing the many scientific shortcomings with the research presented therein, along with the reasons I believe there to be a strong case of scientific fraud against this work. A summary of key issues with the Fisman et al. paper was submitted through the e-submission portal on May 7th, 2022. The attached evaluation of the Fisman et al. publication is in support of my e-submission. It provides additional context and a more in-depth assessment of the serious scientific shortcomings of the study, too many to address within the 3,000-character limit of the online portal.

Of greatest concern is the gross misrepresentation of research findings within the paper and subsequent dissemination by many media outlets of the highly erroneous conclusions of this CMAJ publication. The potential harm of this mis/disinformation on an already divisive society is massive.

I am requesting that the Fisman et al. paper be retracted, immediately. Moreover, given the seriousness of the violations, I am calling on CMAJ to conduct a thorough investigation into this matter and to seek the necessary quality control changes within their organization to ensure published research adheres to established scientific protocols.

If you have any questions or would like to discuss the attached critique in more detail, I can be reached directly at xxx-xxx-xxxx or by email.

Thank you for your attention to this very important matter.

I look forward to your reply.

Sincerely,

Regina Watteel, BSc. Hons Math & Physics, MSc. PhD. Statistics

Email Correspondence

The above letter, couriered to CMAJ on May 12, 2022 was also emailed to the editorial board and CMAJ group on May 16, 2022. In response, CMAJ issued the following form letter.

```
TO: Gena Watteel

FROM: CMAJ Group <cmajgroup@cmaj.ca>

SUBJECT: RE: Attn Kirsten Patrick: Request for Retraction
& Investigation into Scientific Misconduct: CMAJ
2022;194:E573-E580

DATE: May 16, 2022


Dear Regina Watteel,

Thank you for your interest in CMAJ.

We encourage readers who would like to comment on an
article to send a direct letter response to the article
on cmaj.ca.

You can submit your comments by checking the options at
the top of the article page on cmaj.ca (beneath the
article title), where you will see a tab labelled
'Responses'. If you click on it and then on the
hyperlinked text 'Submit a Response to This Article' you
```

will be able to submit your comment.

Almost all e-letters are posted on cmaj.ca and some are later formally published as Letters. Our guidance for authors of e-letters can be found here: https://www.cmaj.ca/content/submitting-letter-editor

Best regards,

Sylvie
Sylvie Blais-Tam
On behalf of the CMAJ Group

TO: CMAJ Group <cmajgroup@cmaj.ca>

CC: Editorial <Editorial@cmaj.ca>

FROM: Gena Watteel

SUBJECT: RE: Attn Kirsten Patrick: Request for Retraction & Investigation into Scientific Misconduct: CMAJ 2022;194:E573-E580

DATE: May 16, 2022

Dear Sylvie,

Thank you for your reply.

I did indeed submit a direct letter response to the article on cmaj.ca on May 7th. I have yet to receive a reply and I am wondering if perhaps the reviewers are overloaded?

Additionally, I attached a thorough critique of the Fisman et al. paper with my email earlier this morning in support of my online submission; the 3000 character limit was not enough to convey all of the issues with the Fisman et al. study.

If you or any of the editors have questions regarding my critique, or would like to discuss this in greater detail, I would be happy to oblige.

Thank you,

Gena
Regina Watteel, BSc. Hons Math & Physics, MSc. PhD. Statistics

Chapter 3

Letters to the University of Toronto

"It was a day when I was preparing a speech to be delivered in praise of the Emperor; there would be a lot of lies in the speech and they would be applauded by those who knew that they were lies."
— Rex Warner, translator, *The Confessions of Saint Augustine*

Three letters were couriered and subsequently emailed to Professor Lori Ferris, the associate Vice-President of Research Oversight and Compliance at the University of Toronto. She was also provided the supplementary document in Appendix A.

In response to the first letter, Professor Ferris claimed that the concerns I raised about the study were not covered under the university's research misconduct framework, and thus not actionable. When I wrote back specifying the exact subsections in the university's framework that dealt with fraud and the willful misrepresentation and misinterpretation of findings, Professor Ferris responded with a fallacious straw man argument. That is, she refuted claims different from the ones I actually made, while pretending not to know the distinction. I sent her a third letter clarifying the allegations for her. She responded by closing the file.

Given the university's conflicts of interest and their behaviour over the course of the pandemic, their reaction to my complaint was not surprising (see *Fisman's Fraud: the Rise of Canadian Hate Science*).

First Letter to University of Toronto & Response

May 26th, 2022
Professor Lori Ferris
Research & Oversight Compliance Office
McMurrich Building, 12 Queen's Park Cresent West, 2nd Floor
Toronto ON, M5S 1S8

CC'd (June 1, 2022): Karen Wallace and the Secretariat on Responsible Conduct of Research

Research Misconduct Submission: David N. Fisman, Ashleigh R. Tuite & Afia Amoako

Dear Professor Lori Ferris and the Research and Oversight Committee:

I have grave concerns regarding the scientific quality, integrity and ethics of the research conducted by Fisman et al. and published by the Canadian Medical Association Journal (CMAJ) on April 25th, 2022:

> David N. Fisman, Afia Amoako, Ashleigh R. Tuite. Impact of population mixing between vaccinated and unvaccinated subpopulations on infectious disease dynamics: implications for SARS-CoV-2 transmission. CMAJ 2022;194:E573-E580

Allegations specific to the University's Framework to Address Allegations of Research Misconduct involve:

> (a) Fraud including the fabrication and falsification of data and results; and
>
> (b) Willfully misrepresenting and misinterpreting findings resulting from conducting research activities.

In short, the Fisman et al. study concocted a model simulation that FLIPPED reality, the authors then asserted their findings as fact and proceeded to inform public policy based on the fabricated results. More specifically, the study leveraged a false premise to support public policy to align with the authors' overt bias against a segment of the population, a bias which is shown to permeate every facet of the study from unsupported opinions to the choice of baseline values, questionable model assumptions, and the misinterpretation of results.

While the modelling itself is wholly inadequate and of extremely poor academic quality, of greatest concern is the gross misrepresentation of research findings within the paper and subsequent dissemination by many media outlets of the highly erroneous conclusions of this University of Toronto study. After publication, the main author continued to push the false narrative through various media channels and has continued to make derogatory and unsubstantiated remarks towards a segment of society. The potential harm of this mis/disinformation on an already divisive society is massive.

I have attached a comprehensive critique of the published study, discussing the many scientific shortcomings with the research presented therein, along with the reasons I believe there to be a **strong case of scientific fraud** against this work. Note that I have submitted a summary of key issues with the Fisman et al. paper to CMAJ through their e-submission portal (within one week of publication rebukes by 22 other scientists and researchers had already been submitted and posted). I have also sent Dr. Kirsten Patrick, CMAJ editor-in-chief, a more thorough evaluation of the Fisman et al. publication and have requested an immediate retraction of the paper. Given the seriousness of the violations, I am now calling on the University of Toronto to conduct a thorough investigation into this matter.

If you have any questions or would like to discuss the attached critique in more detail, I can be reached directly at xxx-xxx-xxxx or by email.

Thank you for your attention to this very important matter.

I look forward to your reply.

Sincerely,

Regina Watteel
BSc. Hons Math & Physics, MSc. PhD. Statistics

UNIVERSITY OF TORONTO RESPONSE

May 31, 2022
Dear Dr. Watteel:

Re: Allegation of Research Misconduct: Afia Amoako, Professor David Fisman, Professor Ashleigh Tuite

I am writing to acknowledge receipt of your correspondence of May 26, 2022.

The University of Toronto responds to allegations of research misconduct under its Policy on Ethical Conduct in Research and its companion Framework to Address Allegations of Research Misconduct (the "Framework"). Research misconduct complaints are reserved for genuine breaches of the integrity of the research process where conduct deviates from the norms of the relevant research community, not honest errors, honest differences in methodology, interpretation or judgement, divergent paradigms in research, or debates of scientific merit. The concerns you have raised in your correspondence are examples of the latter, do not constitute a complaint of research misconduct under the Framework, and are not actionable by the University under the Framework.

You indicated in your correspondence that you raised your concerns with the CMAJ journal through the journal's online portal and via communication to Dr. Kirsten Patrick, the journal's Editor-in-Chief. We encourage the use of academic forums to debate scientific merit.

Sincerely,

Professor Lorraine E. Ferris
Associate Vice President, Research Oversight and Compliance

Second Letter to University of Toronto & Response

June 1st, 2022
Professor Lori Ferris
Research & Oversight Compliance Office
McMurrich Building, 12 Queen's Park Cresent West, 2nd Floor
Toronto ON, M5S 1S8

CC'd: Karen Wallace and the Secretariat on Responsible Conduct of Research

Re: Research Misconduct Submission: David N. Fisman, Ashleigh R. Tuite & Afia Amoako

Dear Professor Lori Ferris and the Research and Oversight Committee:

Thank you for confirming receipt of my formal complaint against David N. Fisman, Ashleigh R. Tuite and Afia Amoako regarding allegations of scientific misconduct.

As specified in my letter, the allegations of fraud and misconduct include fabrication and falsification of data and results as well as willfully misrepresenting and misinterpreting findings resulting from conducting research. Such acts fall well within the University's Framework to Address Allegations of Research Misconduct, as outlined in Section 4.1 (a) and Section 4.1 (m) of the Framework document.

Fabrication and falsification of data and results are two of the most severe violations of research integrity; surely, they are worthy of investigation. Along with my letter of May 26th 2022, I provided a 20-page supporting document that demonstrated clear indications of fraud.

Data fabrication is the act of making up data and reporting the made-up data as a true reflection of events. An example of fabrication includes artificially creating data when it should be collected from an actual experiment[a] or observation, which is exactly what Professor Fisman, Professor Tuite and Afia Amoako did in their study.

Falsification involves a deliberate manipulation of the research process to produce a desired result, including leaving out data that goes against a desired result. Fisman

---
[a] Northern Illinois University, 2022.

et al. concocted a model to generate the results they wanted, completely omitting any reference to readily available real-world data that completely contradicts their results. Then they proceeded to state the contrived results as fact.

Is it the University's position that such acts of fabrication and falsification are the norm in faculty research at the University of Toronto?

These are not frivolous allegations based on a mere difference of opinion, interpretation or judgement. The actions by the authors follow the literal definition of fraud. Moreover, the research errors and misrepresentations do not appear to be honest in nature, as indicated by the words and actions of the main author following publication.

The allegations of misconduct are very serious and the rampant spread of disinformation stemming from the University of Toronto study continues to negatively impact the lives of <u>millions</u> of Canadians. I ask that the University of Toronto reconsider its decision not to take action on this matter as such inaction allows the harm to continue and implicates support or tolerance of the alleged fraud.

If the university chooses not to investigate the matter, they should, at a minimum, request the authors publicly clarify their research findings and set the record straight that their work does not relate to real events – past, present or projected. The main "finding" that people who forgo vaccination contribute disproportionately to risk is unsupported and contrary to real-world observations and must be retracted. Moreover, the authors' unethical assertion that the study supports "public actions aimed at enhancing vaccine uptake and limiting access to public spaces for unvaccinated people" should be denounced by the university as both harmful and erroneous.

Once again, if you have any questions or would like further clarification of the allegations, I can be reached directly at xxx-xxx-xxxx or by email.

I look forward to your reply and reconsideration.

Sincerely,

Regina Watteel
BSc. Hons Math & Physics, MSc. PhD. Statistics

UNIVERSITY OF TORONTO RESPONSE

June 21, 2022
Dear Dr. Watteel:

Re: Allegation of Research Misconduct:
Afia Amoako, Professor David Fisman, Professor Ashleigh Tuite

I am writing in response to your recent correspondence of June 1, 2022.

As indicated in my May 31 letter in response to your May 26th correspondence, the University of Toronto takes research integrity seriously and responds to allegations of research misconduct under its Policy on Ethical Conduct in Research and its companion Framework to Address Allegations of Research Misconduct (the "Framework"). Research misconduct complaints are reserved for genuine breaches of the integrity of the research process where conduct deviates from the norms of the relevant research community, not honest errors, honest differences in methodology, interpretation or judgement, divergent paradigms in research, or debates of scientific merit.

In your June 1st correspondence you state that "fabrication includes artificially creating data when it should be collected from an actual experiment". The Fisman et al paper clearly states that the study is based on a model; this is a well-accepted research methodology and in no way fulfils the criteria for data fabrication. The paper further clearly states the limitations of the model and states that "it does not precisely simulate a real-world pandemic process in all its complexity". Models have value in science even if they cannot mirror the real world with 100% accuracy. The authors' model is publicly available for any interested parties to review, and the merits of the model can be appropriately debated in the scholarly literature through correspondence with the CMAJ. Your further allege that the paper constitutes an example of falsification, as you say that the paper omits real-world data that would contradict the paper's results. The authors have previously responded to similar criticisms regarding the model parameters and their relationship to real-world data on the CMAJ website, and these discussions are important and should be part of the scholarly debate through academic channels, such as the CMAJ. Your allegations are about debates of scientific merit and not research integrity and will not be pursued under the Framework to Address Allegations of Research Misconduct as they are not actionable by the University under the Framework.

Sincerely,

Professor Lorraine E. Ferris
Associate Vice President, Research Oversight and Compliance

Third Letter to U of T, cc'd: CIHR, CMAJ (Clarification of Allegations)

June 26th, 2022
Professor Lori Ferris
Research & Oversight Compliance Office
McMurrich Building, 12 Queen's Park Cresent West, 2nd Floor
Toronto ON, M5S 1S8

Cc: Karen Wallace, Acting Executive Director, Responsible Conduct of Research, CIHR; Kirsten Patrick, Editor-in-Chief, CMAJ

Re: Research Misconduct Submission: David N. Fisman, Ashleigh R. Tuite & Afia Amoako

Dear Professor Lori Ferris and the Research and Oversight Committee:

Thank you for your letter on June 21st which sheds light on your interpretation of the allegations of scientific misconduct against David N. Fisman, Ashleigh R. Tuite and Afia Amoako. I have considered carefully the arguments presented therein and have found that while they provide support for the use of mathematical modelling in science – which is not in question – they do not address, nor provide defense against, the allegations of fraud at hand. I have addressed each of your comments below to further clarify the acts of misconduct at issue in hopes we can reach a satisfactory resolution.

The use of models to simulate hypothetical outcomes and explore real-world phenomenon can, when properly constructed, provide great insight into real-world issues. Such simulations do not, in and of themselves, constitute data fabrication. That is not in dispute. However, passing off simulated data as a true reflection of events without any real-world validation does constitute data fabrication by its very definition. The violation is especially egregious when real-world observations are readily available and such data completely contradicts the contrived results, as in the present case.

Validation of results is a key component of mathematical modelling. It provides a reality-check to ensure the integrity of the findings when making inferences and predictions about real-world scenarios. Moreover, model validation helps eliminate fraud by preventing the complete fabrication of data. That is, validation prevents the kind of fraud we witnessed in the Fisman et al. study where a model is contrived merely to satisfy the highly biased, preconceived notions of the authors.

As you mentioned in your letter, the Fisman et al. paper clearly states that the study is based on a model. However, the fact that a model simulation was the basis for the study in no way negates the need to validate the model and the results before making inferences about real-world outcomes. Indeed, well-established methodology calls for such validation. Certainly, the authors know this since two of them, namely David Fisman and Ashleigh Tuite, specialize in mathematical modelling. Moreover, the main author cites mathematical epidemiology as a primary teaching responsibility.

Yet, no real-world data was modelled. There was no benchmarking or validation of any kind. Hence, no scientifically valid inferences about real-world events are possible from their study. Regardless, the authors go on to state their fabricated results as fact:

> "...we found that the *choices made by people* who forgo vaccination contribute disproportionately to risk among those who do get vaccinated."

> "The **fact** that this excess contribution to risk cannot be mitigated by high like-with-like mixing undermines the assertion that vaccine choice is best left to the individual and **supports strong public actions** aimed at enhancing vaccine uptake and limiting access to public spaces for unvaccinated people, because risk cannot be considered "self-regarding." There is ample precedent for public health regulation that protects the wider community from acquisition of communicable diseases, even if this protection comes at a **cost of individual freedom.**"

The above quotes, taken directly from the Fisman et al. paper, assert a finding regarding choices made by people despite a complete absence of people or real-world observations in their study. They go on to state their findings as fact, falsely claim that their fictitious fact supports "strong public actions" and they even demonstrate awareness that imposing such actions based on their fiction comes at a cost to individual freedom.

Note that the model was not used to project the future, baseline conditions were set to simulate the past. The authors simulated an epidemic that had already occurred this past winter, got it wrong, then proceeded to overwrite history by stating that they "found that the choices made by people who forgo vaccination contribute disproportionately to risk" when, in actuality, incident rates were found to be disproportionately higher amongst vaccinated individuals.

To date, the authors have failed to clarify that their "findings" do not relate to real events and are, in fact, opposite reality. This despite many researchers, scientists and others calling on the authors to do so. Instead, the authors have staunchly stood behind their contrived results to the detriment of society. Concerns provided to CMAJ from fellow researchers have been met with hand-waving dismissive responses, deflections and further falsehoods.

Knowingly stating fiction as fact is fraudulent. Whatever caveats may have been included in the study do not change that. Once brought to the attention of the authors, the journal, and the university, corrections should have been made. Instead, all parties are finding reasons to turn their backs on their duty to uphold scientific integrity thus allowing these false inferences to propagate and cause further harm.

Your letter further justifies inaction by pointing out that the Fisman et al. paper clearly states the limitations of the model. This is not the case as demonstrated by the many issues raised by myself along with other scientists and researchers following the publication. The only weakness mentioned in the paper is that the model "does not precisely simulate a real-world pandemic process in all its complexity" – a statement true of any mathematical model. In true form, the authors go on to provide a single, one-sided example of this weakness, namely that not all the benefits of vaccination were captured. They use this "weakness" to falsely assert that they likely underestimated vaccine benefits, once again without reference to real-world observations that show the opposite.

Far from a declaration of the model's inadequacies, the authors' statement of limitation serves to propel and even magnify the fraudulent results of the study and bolster a political agenda.

You state in your letter that the authors' model is publicly available for any interested parties to review, which I and other researchers have done. Along with my initial letter, I provided a 20-page review of the study that included a number of critical limitations with the contrived model, none of which are mentioned in the Fisman et al. paper. I encourage you to read my review if you haven't done so already; it provides a compelling case of scientific misconduct. I have included it again with this submission, for your convenience.

While I have a strong background in mathematical modelling and can easily recognize the complete invalidity of the research, the erroneous findings were quickly taken up by media and widely distributed to the general public. Is it your view that the onus is on the public to validate findings published by University of Toronto professors? Is it wrong for the average layman to assume that a peer-reviewed study, written by tenured or seasoned professors and published in a Canadian medical journal, had gone through proper scientific rigor – including validation? Certainly, the process isn't perfect and papers slip by that shouldn't. However,

there is an assumption that when egregiously false and harmful findings are brought to the attention of the journal and the research institution, they will be corrected.

As you state, "models have value in science even if they cannot mirror the real world with 100% accuracy." This is certainly true. However, when they fail to adhere to proper scientific methodology they can also be used to mislead. The gross transgressions that allowed for the fraud in the Fisman et al. study are not par for the course. It is not a matter of the model falling short of 100% accuracy. The model they present is both flawed and fraudulent to the point of causing significant societal harm.

One has to be able to distinguish between make-believe and science and there are many tools available to do that. If well-established methodology had been followed, as claimed in your letter, then this fraud would not have survived the process.

I have submitted criticisms of the study to CMAJ. Thus far, only submissions received within one week of the publication date have been posted to their website. I have not been provided information as to if or when the remaining submissions will be posted.

Given the serious nature of these concerns, I notified University of Toronto's Research & Oversight Compliance Office of the allegations and I provided supporting documentation to back up my claims. After receiving the university's initial response to my complaint, I apprised CIHR of the situation. They, along with CMAJ, have been cc'd in this correspondence.

To date, none of my concerns have been sufficiently addressed by the authors nor any of the three institutions involved – CMAJ, University of Toronto, CIHR. I hope this letter provides further clarification into the allegations of misconduct so that the university can thoroughly address all questions presented here and in previous correspondences and work to resolve all concerns as set forth in Sections 6, 7 & 8 of the University's Framework to Address Allegations of Research Misconduct.

As articulated throughout this letter and detailed in previously submitted material, the issues at hand go far beyond debates of scientific merit, they concern fundamental research integrity.

The authors conducted a textbook example of data fabrication and falsification. There is no question their statements of fact are fraudulent with potential for great harm. If this is not worthy of proper investigation, one is left to question what is.

Mathematical modelling does not grant one a license to mislead, to ignore real-world data, to fabricate or falsify results and call them reality. To foster such deception under the guise of science does a disservice to the scientific field, the research institute and to society.

Once again, if you have any questions or would like further clarification of the allegations, I can be reached directly at xxx-xxx-xxxx or by email.

I look forward to a thorough response to my many questions and concerns and to a satisfactory resolution.

Sincerely,

Regina Watteel
BSc. Hons Math & Physics, MSc. PhD. Statistics

R.N. Watteel, PhD Statistics

University of Toronto Final Response & Decision

July 19, 2022

Dear Dr. Watteel:

Re: Allegation of Research Misconduct:
Afia Amoako, Professor David Fisman, Professor Ashleigh Tuite

I am writing in response to your correspondence of June 27, 2022.

Your letter of June 27 did not raise anything new that we did not address in our May 31 and June 21 communication to you.

Therefore, nothing from your submission is actionable under the Framework to Address Allegations of Research Misconduct.

The University's file on this matter is closed.

Sincerely,

Professor Lorraine E. Ferris
Associate Vice President, Research Oversight and Compliance

CHAPTER 4
Letters to CIHR

"It takes two things to make a political lie work: a powerful person or institution willing to utter it, and another set of powerful institutions to amplify it."
— Eric S. Perlstein, American historian and journalist (1969-)

The Canadian Institutes of Health Research (CIHR) is the federal institution that funded the Fisman et al. study. CIHR is accountable to Parliament through the Minister of Health. CIHR's Secretariat on Responsible Conduct of Research claims to be interested in ensuring the public record is correct, reliable and accurate.[b]

On June 1, 2022 CIHR was sent a letter apprising them that a complaint of research misconduct had been filed with the University of Toronto against David Fisman, Ashleigh Tuite and Afia Amoako. They were also provided a full complement of supporting documentation, including the document in Appendix A and the letters that had been written to, and received by, the university in regards to the complaint. Once the university closed the case without addressing any of the concerns raised, I filed a complaint with CIHR against the University of Toronto for breach of the Tri-Agency Research Integrity Policy.

Despite the solid evidence against the researchers and the university,

---
[b] Collier, Roger, 2015.

the manner in which the falsities were propagated by the media and used by members of Parliament to justify harmful restrictions against the unvaccinated, the Agency Presidents decided not to take corrective action.

Letter to CIHR: Misconduct Allegations

June 1st, 2022
Secretariat on Responsible Conduct of Research
Canadian Institutes of Health Research
160 Elgin Street, 9th Floor
Ottawa ON K1A 0W9
Canada

Complaint of Research Misconduct: David N. Fisman, Ashleigh R. Tuite & Afia Amoako

Dear Karen Wallace and the Secretariat on Responsible Conduct of Research (SRCR):

This letter is to advise the SRCR that I have filed a complaint with the University of Toronto regarding the scientific quality, integrity and ethics of the research conducted by Fisman et al., funded by the Canadian Institutes of Health Research (CIHR)[c] and published by the Canadian Medical Association Journal (CMAJ) on April 25th, 2022:

> David N. Fisman, Afia Amoako, Ashleigh R. Tuite. Impact of population mixing between vaccinated and unvaccinated subpopulations on infectious disease dynamics: implications for SARS-CoV-2 transmission. CMAJ 2022;194:E573-E580

The allegations of fraud and misconduct include fabrication and falsification of data and results as well as willfully misrepresenting and misinterpreting findings resulting from conducting research.

---

[c] The research was supported by a grant to David Fisman; 2019 COVID-19 rapid researching funding OV4-170360.

Despite the fact that fabrication and falsification of data and results are two of the most severe violations of research integrity and that such acts fall well within the University's Framework to Address Allegations of Research Misconduct, the University of Toronto initially declined to take action. I have since asked the university to reconsider (please see email correspondence below).

Along with my initial letter to the university, I provided a 20-page supporting document that clearly demonstrates the allegations of fraud. I've attached the document to this email for your review along with my formal letters to Professor Lori Ferris at the Research & Oversight Compliance Office, University of Toronto.

The allegations of misconduct are very serious and the rampant spread of disinformation stemming from the Fisman et al. study continues to negatively impact the lives of millions of Canadians. I ask that CIHR look into this matter to ensure it is treated with due diligence.

If you have any questions or would like further clarification of the allegations, I can be reached directly at xxx-xxx-xxxx or by email.

I look forward to your reply and consideration.

Sincerely,

Regina Watteel
BSc. Hons Math & Physics, MSc. PhD. Statistics

Letter to CIHR: Breach of Policy by UofT

July 25th, 2022
Secretariat on Responsible Conduct of Research
Canadian Institutes of Health Research
160 Elgin Street, 9th Floor
Ottawa ON K1A 0W9
Canada

ACTION REQUIRED: Breach of Tri-Agency Research Integrity Policy by University of Toronto

Dear Karen Wallace and the Secretariat on Responsible Conduct of Research (SRCR):

This letter serves to update the SRCR on what has transpired since my initial correspondence on June 1st, 2022 regarding a complaint of research misconduct filed with the University of Toronto against David N. Fisman, Afia Amoako and Ashleigh R. Tuite. The work in question was funded by the Canadian Institutes of Health Research (CIHR)[1] and published in the Canadian Medical Association Journal (CMAJ) on April 25th, 2022[2].

The acts of misconduct include fabrication and falsification of data and results as well as willfully misrepresenting and misinterpreting findings resulting from conducting research. The fraudulent work has been used to inform government policy; the influence of the study and its authors is ongoing.

This letter is to advise SRCR that the University of Toronto has failed in its duty to address this serious allegation of research misconduct in breach of its commitment to CIHR under Section 4.2a of the Tri-Agency Responsible Conduct of Research Framework. Given the serious nature of the misconduct and its far-reaching implications, this matter requires immediate attention and action by SRCR.

Background:

On May 26th, 2022 a complaint was filed with the University of Toronto regarding a fraudulent study authored by tenured professor David N. Fisman and two of his colleagues, Afia Amoako and Ashleigh R. Tuite. A 20-page supporting document detailing the study's lack of scientific merit and research integrity was provided. This document included specific examples of fraudulent assertions made by the authors as well the harmful implications thereof.

On May 31st, 2022 I received a response from Professor Lorraine E. Ferris, Associate Vice President Research Oversight and Compliance U of T, regarding my initial request for an investigation into the allegations. Professor Ferris stated that my concerns of fraud, including falsification and fabrication, did not constitute a complaint of research misconduct under the university's Framework to Address Allegations of Research Misconduct (the "Framework"). However, Section 4.1 (a) and Section 4.1 (m) of the Framework indicate otherwise. More troubling, the response suggested that such conduct was within the norms of the relevant research community at the university.

To clarify any misinterpretation, I sent a follow-up letter to Professor Ferris on June 1st, 2022 specifying the exact violations under the Framework and providing references that demonstrate the acts of misconduct by Fisman et al. are indeed recognized as acts of fraud in the research community. It was at that time that I informed SRCR of the complaint filed with the University of Toronto against Fisman et al. All correspondence with the university was provided to SRCR, including the 20-page document supporting the allegations.

On June 21st, I received a rather terse letter from Professor Ferris addressing claims that were not made in the complaint I had filed while skirting the very serious acts of misconduct in question. The letter indicated that either (1) the Associate VP of Research Oversight and Compliance had a complete lack of knowledge regarding the difference between what constitutes well-accepted research methodology in the field of mathematical modelling and what constitutes a textbook case of scientific fraud, or (2) her office had no intention of giving this matter the due consideration they are obliged to under the Framework.

To further clarify, on June 26th I provided my third letter to Professor Ferris that addressed each point she raised, thus nullifying any attempt to deflect from the true nature of the complaint against Fisman et al. SRCR was cc'd in the correspondence. Indeed, this third and final letter eliminated any excuse for inaction and presented a damning indictment of the university's decision not to investigate.

The Fisman et al. study is an egregious act of research misconduct with potential for great societal harm that requires a proper investigation. Failure to do so indicates complicity in the fraud.

On July 19th, 2022 I received final confirmation that the university had chosen to renege on their commitment to research integrity. They refused to take this complaint of gross misconduct seriously. Professor Ferris's letter was short and to the point: "The University's file on this matter is closed."

Instead of investigating the allegations, seeking advice from a colleague knowledgeable in the field of mathematical modelling, or, at the very least, asking the researchers to correct and clarify their false assertions, Dr. Ferris closed the file. _Not a single concern had been addressed._

Professor Ferris's handling of the case is in violation of Sections 6, 7 & 8 of the University's Framework. That is, the University of Toronto did not adhere to its own research conduct policy as required in Section 4.2a of the Tri-Agency Responsible Conduct of Research Framework.

Societal Impact - Urgency:

The work by Fisman et al. failed to adhere to even the most basic research and ethics protocols, including breaches in Tri-Agency research integrity policies Sections 3.1.1.a (fabrication) and 3.1.1.b (falsification).

Over a dozen rebukes submitted by 22 researchers and health care professionals were brought to the attention of the researchers and posted on the CMAJ website within one-week of the study's publication. The authors acknowledged that they had received criticism regarding their incorrect interpretation of model results along with concerns that their model is stoking hatred. Instead of taking proper action and clarifying their findings, the researchers have staunchly stood behind their contrived results to the detriment of society.

Not only were the falsified findings quickly taken up and disseminated by numerous media outlets nationwide in a publicity blitz, one week after publication the study was waived around in Parliament by Liberal MP Adam van Koeverden, citing it as justification for extending travel restrictions against the unvaccinated.

Clearly, such fraudulent methods cannot be permitted to influence policy and sow societal division. And while travel restrictions and vaccine mandates have been suspended for the moment, threats of reinstating them loom so long as such fraudulent and scientifically baseless claims against the unvaccinated population are permitted to stand.

Actions Requested:

The failure of CMAJ and U of T to address this serious matter is indicative of an institutional resistance to <u>self-correct and learn from the pandemic</u>. This shortcoming is costly to public health, the economy and to social cohesion. It stifles progress and erodes trust in our health and research institutions. We need to move forward in a more positive, comprehensive and beneficial manner.

In order to remedy the wrongdoing, I respectfully request the following actions be taken by CIHR:

1. Issue a letter of concern to the main researcher David N. Fisman.

2. Request the authors retract their CMAJ publication[2].

3. Request that the researchers make a public statement clarifying their research findings and set the record straight that their work does not relate to real events – past, present or projected. The main "finding" that people who forgo vaccination contribute disproportionately to risk is <u>unsupported and contrary</u> to real-world observations and must be

retracted.

4. Notify Parliament of the fraud and inform members that the study findings presented in the House of Commons on April 29th, 2022 by Liberal MP Adam van Koeverden, Parliamentary Secretary to the Minister of Health, were erroneous and in fact contrary to real-world data.[3] The study does not, in actuality, provide any scientific support for "public actions aimed at enhancing vaccine uptake and limiting access to public spaces for unvaccinated people" nor does it support any other restriction against those who are not vaccinated.

5. The researchers' credibility is clearly compromised in this area and this brings into question any previous work, recommendations, and advocacy these researchers have conducted regarding the pandemic. As such, it is advisable that:

a. All relevant public institutions and agencies be notified of the fraud[4];

b. All such work funded by CIHR be reviewed for errors and bias, especially in regards to Covid-19 vaccination or anything derived from mathematical modelling exercises done in part, wholly, or influenced by any of the three researchers; and,

c. The Agency not accept applications for future funding from the researchers in relation to the Covid-19 pandemic.

If you have any questions or would like further clarification of the allegations, I can be reached directly at xxx-xxx-xxxx or by email.

I ask that you confirm receipt of this letter.

I look forward to your reply and consideration.

Sincerely,

Regina Watteel
BSc. Hons Math & Physics, MSc. PhD. Statistics

Email Correspondence with CIHR

TO: secretariat <secretariat@srcr-scrr.gc.ca>, karen.wallace <karen.wallace@srcr-scrr.gc.ca>

FROM: Gena Watteel

SUBJECT: ACTION REQUIRED: Breach of Tri-Agency Research Integrity Policy by University of Toronto

DATE: Jul 25, 2022, 11:50 AM

Dear Karen Wallace and the Secretariat on Responsible Conduct of Research (SRCR):

This letter serves to update the SRCR on what has transpired since my initial correspondence on June 1st, 2022 regarding a complaint of research misconduct filed with the University of Toronto against David N. Fisman, Afia Amoako and Ashleigh R. Tuite. The work in question was funded by the Canadian Institutes of Health Research (CIHR)[1] and published in the Canadian Medical Association Journal (CMAJ) on April 25th, 2022[2].

The acts of misconduct include fabrication and falsification of data and results as well as willfully misrepresenting and misinterpreting findings resulting from conducting research. The fraudulent work has been used to inform government policy; the influence of the study and its authors is ongoing.

This letter is to advise SRCR that the University of Toronto has failed in its duty to address this serious allegation of research misconduct in breach of its commitment to CIHR under Section 4.2a of the Tri-Agency Responsible Conduct of Research Framework. Given the serious nature of the misconduct and its far-reaching implications, <u>this matter requires immediate attention and action by SRCR</u>.

The following documents are attached to this email:

1. SRCR_Breach of Policy by UT 2022-07-25.pdf: A letter explaining the breach, all communications with the University of Toronto in regards to the allegations of misconduct, and the actions sought from SRCR.

2. Signed Research Misconduct Letter 3_Fisman Study.pdf: The third and final letter provided to University of Toronto and cc'd to SRCR on June 26th clarifying the allegations of misconduct;

3. Supporting documentation Reseach Misconduct Fisman et al.pdf: The 20-page supporting document detailing the acts of research misconduct that was provided to the University of Toronto and SRCR.

If you have any questions or would like to discuss this matter in person or by phone, I can be reached directly at xxx-xxx-xxxx or by email.

I look forward to your response and timely action on this matter.

Sincerely,

Regina Watteel
BSc. Hons Math & Physics, MSc. PhD. Statistics

TO: Gena Watteel

FROM: Wallace, Karen (SRCR/SCRR) <Karen.Wallace@srcr-scrr.gc.ca>

SUBJECT: FW: ACTION REQUIRED: Breach of Tri-Agency Research Integrity Policy by University of Toronto

DATE: Aug 18, 2022, 1:30 PM

Hello Dr. Watteel,

The Secretariat acknowledges receipt of your July 25, 2022 email below, as well as other documents that you sent to its office by mail, regarding your allegation against the University of Toronto in addressing your complaint of research misconduct against Dr. David Fisman et al.

In order for the Secretariat to move forward regarding your allegation of breach of the RCR Framework by the University of Toronto, we are requesting your permission to share the attached July 25th letter with the responsible conduct of research contact at the University of Toronto, Dr. Lorraine Ferris, so that they have an opportunity to respond to your concern.

Once we receive the University's response, the Secretariat will determine next steps and inform you of them in a timely manner.

Regards,

Karen Wallace

A/Executive Director

Secretariat on Responsible Conduct of Research / Government of Canada

karen.wallace@srcr-scrr.gc.ca / Tel: 343-552-3119

TO: Wallace, Karen (SRCR/SCRR) <Karen.Wallace@srcr-scrr.gc.ca>

FROM: Gena Watteel

SUBJECT: Re: FW: ACTION REQUIRED: Breach of Tri-Agency Research Integrity Policy by University of Toronto

DATE: Aug 19, 2022, 10:29 AM

Hi Karen,

Thank you for looking into this very serious matter. Yes, please feel free to share the July 25th letter with Dr. Lorraine Ferris.

I look forward to hearing about the Secretariat's next steps.

Kind regards,

Regina Watteel
BSc. Hons Math & Physics, MSc. PhD. Statistics

TO: Wallace, Karen (SRCR/SCRR) <Karen.Wallace@srcr-scrr.gc.ca>

FROM: Gena Watteel

SUBJECT: Re: FW: ACTION REQUIRED: Breach of Tri-Agency Research Integrity Policy by University of Toronto

DATE: Sep 22, 2022, 10:18 AM

Hi Karen,

I'm just following up on the status of the University of Toronto policy breach and the misconduct allegations against Dr. Fisman et al.

Has there been any progress?

Thank you kindly,

Regina Watteel
BSc. Hons Math & Physics, MSc. PhD. Statistics

TO: Wallace, Karen (SRCR/SCRR) <Karen.Wallace@srcr-scrr.gc.ca>

FROM: Gena Watteel

SUBJECT: Re: FW: ACTION REQUIRED: Breach of Tri-Agency Research Integrity Policy by University of Toronto

DATE: Oct 11, 2022, 11:30 AM

Hi Karen,

Could you please provide me with a status update regarding the University of Toronto policy breach and the misconduct allegations against Fisman et al?

It has been almost five months since I first contacted the university and requested an investigation into the fraudulent study written by David N. Fisman, Afia Amoako and Ashleigh R. Tuite. Their highly publicized study continues to be referenced thus compounding its negative impacts.

Thank you kindly,

Regina Watteel
BSc. Hons Math & Physics, MSc. PhD. Statistics

TO: secretariat@srcr-scrr.gc.ca

Cc: Wallace, Karen (SRCR/SCRR) <Karen.Wallace@srcr-scrr.gc.ca>

FROM: Gena Watteel

SUBJECT: Fwd: FW: ACTION REQUIRED: Breach of Tri-Agency Research Integrity Policy by University of Toronto

DATE: Oct 24, 2022, 12:25 PM

Dear Secretariat on Responsible Conduct of Research (SRCR):

I am seeking a status update regarding the University of Toronto policy breach and the misconduct allegations against Fisman et al.

On several occasions I have reached out to SRCR (Karen Wallace) to provide such an update and have yet to receive a response. I have included the email correspondence below.

I would very much appreciate an update on this file and I thank you for looking into this matter.

Regina Watteel
BSc. Hons Math & Physics, MSc. PhD. Statistics

TO: Gena Watteel

FROM: Wallace, Karen (SRCR/SCRR) <Karen.Wallace@srcr-scrr.gc.ca>

SUBJECT: RE: FW: ACTION REQUIRED: Breach of Tri-Agency Research Integrity Policy by University of Toronto

DATE: Oct 24, 2022, 3:55 PM

Hello Dr. Watteel,

My apologies for the delay in responding to your emails below.

Your allegations against the University of Toronto and the University's response to them were considered by the Panel on Responsible Conduct of Research last month. The next step in the RCR process is for the matter to be considered by the Presidents of the Agencies for final decision. A final decision on this matter is expected before the end of November 2022.

The Secretariat will inform you of the final decision at that time.

Regards,

Karen Wallace

A/Executive Director

Secretariat on Responsible Conduct of Research / Government of Canada

karen.wallace@srcr-scrr.gc.ca / Tel: 343-552-3119

TO: Wallace, Karen (SRCR/SCRR) <Karen.Wallace@srcr-scrr.gc.ca>

FROM: Gena Watteel

SUBJECT: RE: FW: ACTION REQUIRED: Breach of Tri-Agency Research Integrity Policy by University of Toronto

DATE: Oct 24, 2022, 4:56 PM

Much appreciated. Thank you!

Regina Watteel

TO: Wallace, Karen (SRCR/SCRR) <Karen.Wallace@srcr-scrr.gc.ca>

FROM: Gena Watteel

SUBJECT: Re: FW: ACTION REQUIRED: Breach of Tri-Agency Research Integrity Policy by University of Toronto

DATE: Dec 5, 2022, 8:30 AM

Good Morning Karen.

Back in October, you had mentioned that a final decision regarding the University of Toronto policy breach and the misconduct allegations against Fisman et al. was expected by the end of November. Have the Presidents of the Agencies reached a decision?

Either way, I would like to schedule an in-person meeting with either the Panel on Responsible Conduct of Research or the Presidents of the Agencies to discuss this further. Is it possible to set something up in the next couple of weeks, preferably before Christmas?

Thank you kindly,

Regina Watteel
BSc. Hons Math & Physics, MSc. PhD. Statistics

TO: Gena Watteel

FROM: Wallace, Karen (SRCR/SCRR) <Karen.Wallace@srcr-scrr.gc.ca>

SUBJECT: RE: FW: ACTION REQUIRED: Breach of Tri-Agency Research Integrity Policy by University of Toronto

DATE: Dec 9, 2022, 10:34 AM

Hello Dr. Watteel,

A final decision has recently been made by the Presidents of the Agencies related to your allegation that the University of Toronto breached article 4.2(a) of the Tri-Agency Framework: Responsible Conduct of Research (RCR Framework). You and the University of Toronto will be informed of that decision shortly.

Neither the Presidents nor the Panel are in a position to meet with parties associated with research misconduct allegations as it is not part of the Agencies' process for addressing allegations of breach of the RCR Framework. If you need information on the Agencies' process apart from what appears in the RCR Framework, the Secretariat is prepared to speak with you by MS Teams.

Regards,

Karen Wallace

Executive Director

Secretariat on Responsible Conduct of Research / Government of Canada

karen.wallace@srcr-scrr.gc.ca / Tel: 343-552-3119

FINAL DECISION

TO: Gena Watteel

FROM: Wallace, Karen (SRCR/SCRR) <Karen.Wallace@srcr-scrr.gc.ca>

SUBJECT: Correspondence from SRCR

DATE: Dec 19, 2022, 4:40 PM

Dear Dr. Watteel,

The RCR process regarding your allegation of institutional non-compliance against the University of Toronto has concluded. The Agencies Presidents have determined that the University complied with Article 4.2(a) of the Tri-Agency Framework: Responsible Conduct of Research when addressing the allegations that you made against Dr. Fisman et al. The University conducted an inquiry and concluded that your allegations against Dr. Fisman et al. fell within the realm of scientific debate. As noted by the University in its correspondence to you, scientific debate is important, but allegations of breach of Agency or institutional policy are not the appropriate mechanism for addressing differences of scholarly opinion. The Agency Presidents agree.

Our file on this matter is closed.

Regards,

Karen Wallace

Executive Director

Secretariat on Responsible Conduct of Research / Government of Canada

karen.wallace@srcr-scrr.gc.ca / Tel: 343-552-3119

TO: Wallace, Karen (SRCR/SCRR) <Karen.Wallace@srcr-scrr.gc.ca>

FROM: Gena Watteel

SUBJECT: Re: Correspondence from SRCR

DATE: Dec 20, 2022, 7:31 PM

Dear Karen Wallace and the Secretariat on Responsible Conduct of Research (SRCR):

As disappointing as this decision is, I would like to thank you for confirming CIHR's active involvement in what appears to be blatant fraud and hate science levied against Canadians.

I implore you to reopen the case and reconsider.

Sincerely,
Regina Watteel
BSc. Hons Math & Physics, MSc. PhD. Statistics

Chapter 5
Letter to Ontario Premier Ford

"The most dangerous man to any government is the man who is able to think things out for himself, without regard to the prevailing superstitions and taboos."
— Henry Louis Mencken, American Journalist (1880-1956)

By the fall of 2022, there were strong indications that CIHR was likely to sweep Fisman et al.'s misconduct under the rug. Months passed with no update, emails went unanswered, decisions delayed. Then, in the final week before Christmas 2022, their dismissal of the allegations was confirmed.

Each time an institution that claimed to value research integrity decided instead to turn a blind eye to the overt fraud, I dug a little deeper. *What potential interest did they have in the perpetuation of the faux COVID-19 transmission narrative?* By the time CIHR alerted me of their decision to ignore the scientific fraud and allow the public record to go uncorrected, a much larger network of malfeasance had become apparent.

Having anticipated CIHR's response, I had already begun drafting a detailed report to the OPP. On February 5, 2023 I couriered a comprehensive 150-page evidentiary report to OPP Commissioner Thomas Carrique, along with an accompanying letter requesting an investigation. I also couriered Premier Ford the material and asked that he support an OPP investigation.

The cover letter to the premier is presented below (lightly redacted). My dealings with the OPP were much more involved and confirmed the need to explore alternative channels in order to correct the public record and prevent more harm from accruing. The result: *Fisman's Fraud: the Rise of Canadian Hate Science* was forged.

Letter to Premier Ford

Feb 3, 2023
Doug Ford
Premier of Ontario
Legislative Building
Queen's Park
Toronto, ON M7A 1A1

Dear Doug Ford:

I am writing to you today to apprise you of serious acts of fraud relating to COVID-19 pandemic research that involve a prominent researcher, David Fisman, and two of his colleagues, Afia Amoako and Ashleigh R. Tuite. Dr. Fisman has been both outspoken and influential in shaping Ontario's pandemic response. Despite numerous conflicts of interest, he took on several COVID-19 advisory roles and served on the Ontario Covid-19 Science Advisory Table.

The evidence against the three perpetrators is irrefutable, impacting millions of Canadians. I have written several letters to CMAJ, University of Toronto and CIHR detailing the misconduct and seeking a retraction of the paper. I now believe there is sufficient evidence to make the case for (fraud). Given the far-reaching implications of the duplicitous research and the main author's continued influence in pandemic response, I have requested the OPP conduct (an investigation) into these acts. I have included the letter and materials I sent to OPP Commissioner Thomas Carrique that detail the allegations and evidence gathered.

The accompanying material clearly indicates that the authors' credibility in regards to COVID-19 has been compromised. This brings into question any previous work, recommendations, and advocacy these authors have conducted regarding the pandemic, including any work done for the Ontario government. As such, I am

asking that you support an investigation into this matter.

I look forward to your response. I can be reached directly at (xxx) xxx-xxxx or by email.

Sincerely,

Regina Watteel
BSc. Hons. Math & Physics, MSc. PhD. Statistics

APPENDIX A
Critique of CMAJ Study

Fisman et al. SARS-Cov-2 population mixing study FLIPS reality to inform policy and punish the unvaccinated.

Summary

The recent paper by Fisman et al., 2022 "sought to explore the impact of mixing of vaccinated and unvaccinated populations on risk of SARS-Cov-2 infection among vaccinated people." To this end, the authors developed a simple deterministic model to simulate **hypothetical** outcomes of incident cases in Ontario Canada[d] under various group mixing scenarios. The model itself is wholly inadequate, poorly constructed, baseline conditions vaguely specified, key parameters and classifications poorly defined, model assumptions highly biased and the interpretation of their results fundamentally flawed.

 The authors make no attempt to test their model or to reconcile the obvious discrepancy between the incidence rates produced by their model and the actual incidence rates observed during the Dec. 2021 – Jan. 2022 epidemic wave, the first true test of the vaccination strategy in Canada. In

---

[d] As indicated in Table 1 of Fisman et al. 2022

fact, the authors don't mention this outbreak at all. Incredulously, the authors then proceed to use the *simulated outcomes* from their modelling exercise as a basis to inform public policy whilst *failing to even recognize the necessity of looking at the actual real-world outcomes!* A quick visit to the Ontario Covid-19 website[e] uncovers a stark contrast between reality and the authors' "findings." Indeed, the simulated results are *opposite* to the reality that played out in Ontario during the Dec/Jan epidemic wave.

At its core, the population mixing paper written by David N. Fisman, Afia Amoako and Ashleigh R. Tuite appears to be scientific fiction: The authors concoct an unrealistic model to explore the impact of assortative mixing on disease dynamics and contribution to risk and then attempt to pass off the fictitious findings as *fact* in order to inform policy that seeks to unjustly vilify and violate the rights of individuals who forgo covid vaccination.

The complete lack of scientific quality and integrity is truly astounding, especially coming from a tenured professor of epidemiology (the main author) who highlights mathematical modelling & simulation along with decision analysis & cost-effectiveness analysis as research interests. While numerous scientists rebuked the study and its "findings,"[5] the concerns go far beyond poor-quality model building and a mere misinterpretation of results. How the study's many shortcomings escaped the journals peer-review process is unfathomable. Indeed, concerns of bias, falsification, fabrication, misrepresentation, inappropriate influence, and potential political interference are not to be taken lightly.

The highly erroneous "findings" of this University of Toronto study were quickly taken up and disseminated by over a dozen media outlets in the country and have received international coverage. In addition, the paper has been misused and the findings misrepresented – entities in the oversimplified simulation have been dangerously equated to flesh-and-blood people and the applicability of the study was made out to be current day despite its results being in stark contrast to observed trends. This has resulted in the propagation of fear, mistrust, and derisive attitudes towards a segment of the population in the real world who bear absolutely no resemblance to the entities in Fisman et al.'s model. The potential harm of this mis/disinformation on an already divisive society is

---

[e] Ontario.ca. "COVID-19 cases by vaccination status." Accesssed March 10, 2022. https://covid-19.ontario.ca/data#vaccinationStatus4Eligible

massive.

Given the seriousness of the offences and the influence of the authors, this matter warrants a thorough investigation by the University of Toronto. It is prudent to consider strict disciplinary measures to counter both the societal harm of the study and the potential long-term reputational harm on the university that may well follow once an apolitical, retrospective assessment of the pandemic is possible.

Below is a brief overview of <u>*some*</u> of the major issues with the study together with the true implications of the research put forth by Fisman et al., as well as the reasons I believe there to be a strong case of scientific fraud against this work.

Concern #1: Overt Bias

The authors' overt bias, which heavily favors vaccination, permeates every facet of this study from unsupported opinions to the choice of baseline values, questionable model assumptions, and the misinterpretation of results. The bias even extends beyond this scope to inappropriately and irresponsibly inform public policy.

The paper commences with praise regarding vaccine development while disparaging comments regarding disinformation are pointedly directed at the contrarian (so called "antivaccine") sentiment along with a broad statement about the harms of such information, mainly due to decreased vaccine uptake. There is no mention of the many pro-vaccine claims that have proven false over the past year, nor is there mention of the organized coercive tactics that have been used to increase vaccine uptake nor their potential harm or unintended consequences. The authors go on to make false comparisons between choosing not to vaccinate and reckless behavior such as driving under the influence of alcohol and other intoxicants.

The inclusion of unnecessary, subjective opinions in the study's introduction sets the stage for the slanted modelling that follows. The propaganda then returns in the interpretation section of the paper where the authors blame the "unvaccinated" (a classification term they didn't even bother to define) for poor policy decisions made by our public health care system that led to the cancellation of elective surgeries for cancer and cardiac disease. Indeed, if vaccinated individuals cannot get the care they need, the authors put blame squarely on the unvaccinated.[6]

These outrageous and completely baseless claims have no place in what should be an <u>objective</u> scientific paper. The unsupported comments are a strong indication that the authors are ready to inject their personal beliefs into the study rather than perform the tasks required to produce objective research.

Indeed, the modelling itself is riddled with bias. For example, vaccine effectiveness is overstated[7] and waning immunity amongst the vaccinated is completely ignored whilst natural immunity is understated.[8] Both vaccine effectiveness and natural immunity amongst the unvaccinated are key inputs, so any bias passes directly through to the model outputs and results including the so-called attack rates (used to justify segregating the population), and the dubiously defined ψ (used to assign transmission blame).

Even the purported limitation section of the paper demonstrates an inability to recognize bias and properly assess the many model shortcomings. The only "weakness" mentioned is that the model "does not precisely simulate a real-world pandemic process" and thus they likely (substantially) underestimated vaccine benefits.[9] A quick crosscheck against real-world data proves this notion entirely false, in fact opposite, as explained in later sections.

Concern #2: Poorly constructed, inadequate modelling

Perhaps the most important shortcoming of this modelling exercise is that it lacks any meaningful hypothesis or model fitting. To be clear:

- **<u>No hypothesis is being tested</u>** and **<u>no observational data is modelled</u>** in this study, therefore **no meaningful inferences can be drawn** about the real-world impact of population mixing regarding SARS-CoV-2 transmission.

- **This is not a factual study**. This is a HYPOTHETICAL exercise, and a poorly drafted one at that. The model is exploratory in nature with absolutely **no benchmarking or validation of any kind**. Simplistic models in this class are generally not to be taken seriously.

As noted by the authors, simple mathematical models can provide important insights into the behaviour of complex communicable diseases when done properly. Unfortunately, as demonstrated by the authors, when fundamental scientific standards are ignored, these models can lead to hugely erroneous conclusions and stifle progress. More on this in the next section.

As discussed previously, the study demonstrated a complete lack of scientific objectivity and this shortcoming filtered through to all aspects of model building. In addition to this critical flaw, there were several other glaring shortcomings. The most obvious modelling deficiencies are listed below.

A. The use of a deterministic model to simulate a highly stochastic process

Pandemic conditions are dynamic and the SARS-Cov-2 virus is constantly mutating. Vaccine efficacy and immunity depend on a multitude of factors and conditions, many of which change over time. Risk of infection and transmission change depending on the prevailing viral strain and population incidence rates. These fluid conditions bring about a great deal of uncertainty that must be incorporated into any serious model in order to draw meaningful inferences. Moreover, because risk of infection depends on age, underlying health, environmental factors etc., community incidence and transmission will to some extent be impacted by regional factors such as demographics, population density, climate/season etc. As such, establishing a well-defined modelling baseline is also essential.

The model outcomes are probabilistic in nature. Not only must initial conditions be specified, the uncertainties in the input parameters MUST be reflected in the modelling in order to provide meaningful results along with a measure of confidence in those results. We are dealing with a highly dynamic stochastic process and that requires _stochastic_ modelling.

Fisman et al.'s simple model fails to account for many key factors driving transmission and fails to capture realistic transmission dynamics. The authors of the study also fail to acknowledge that uncertainty equates to risk and thus any discussion about risk must incorporate uncertainty.

B. Ambiguous terms, poorly constructed model parameters, unsupported baseline estimates, misuse of basic terminology:

- The authors did not specify the criteria for classifying individuals as unvaccinated or vaccinated (does the "vaccinated" group include partially vaccinated, two doses, three doses...).

- It is unclear how authors chose the baseline values of 0.4 and 0.8 for vaccine effectiveness; the values appear to be arbitrary (i.e. "guesstimates"). A brief discussion of how these values were chosen or derived from the range of estimates provided in the papers referenced by the authors would be helpful, especially in light of the fact that vaccine effectiveness depends on which vaccine an individual takes and time since last dose. What assumptions are the authors using in setting their baseline values?

- The baseline immunity imparted by the vaccines are over-estimated based on literature and without the incorporation of waning immunity this bias is further augmented (Chemaitelly et al., 2021). There seems to be no basis for the low baseline value of 0.2 for immunity within the unvaccinated population (Majdoubi et al. 2021). These deficiencies are not minor. They drive the results.

- The concept of uncertainty seems to have escaped the authors. The authors did not incorporate any meaningful measure of uncertainty in their deterministic model. The authors state: "Our lower-bound estimate for vaccine effectiveness (40%) reflected uncertainty about the emerging Omicron variant." A point estimate is not an incorporation of uncertainty. While the authors run a series of hypothetical scenarios in an attempt to capture the reduced effectiveness of vaccines to emerging variants, this range doesn't reflect the true uncertainty of the estimates where vaccine effectiveness values dip below zero depending on time since last vaccination.[6]

- Failure to capture waning immunity and to adequately model transmission dynamics (serious flaws): "We treated immunity after vaccination as an all-or-none phenomenon, with a fraction of vaccinated people (as defined by vaccine effectiveness) entering the model in the immune state and the remainder being left in the susceptible state."[1] While the authors refer to their model as simple, a better word would be inadequate, evidenced by its failure to even represent the real-world results in its spectrum of possibilities.

- The authors construct a dubious output measure, ψ, which they interpret as the degree to which risk in one group may be disproportionately driven by contact with another. No information is provided about the reliability or validity of this newly constructed measure. Its interpretation is by no means transparent; it requires greater scientific scrutiny before being accepted as meaningful.

- The true driver of incidence rates is immunity not vaccination. There are many factors that weigh into an individual's immunity and risk of infection including: previous infection, overall health of the individual, age, vocation, vaccination status, type of vaccine administered and time since last dose etc. The fact that the authors focus on one, highly political factor to inform public policy suggests a politically motivated agenda or bias. Wouldn't a more positive approach advocate for a healthy lifestyle that builds up one's immunity? Focus on overall health would help reduce illness and disease across the board, not just covid outcomes.

- It is worth discussing what categories should be defined in order to inform policy: e.g. vaccinated versus unvaccinated or immune versus not immune or high risk versus low risk. For example, when modelling the Omicron case, the immunity values were set to 0.2 for the unvaccinated group and 0.4 for the vaccinated group. Ignoring for a moment that this is opposite the pattern of observed incidence rates, surely such arbitrary values must be assigned a high degree of uncertainty. An uncertainty of merely 0.1 on the same scale for each group produces the possibility for overlap. Thus, immunity could be granted to the same proportion of entities for each group, and yet one group is to be severely penalized with travel bans and mandates while the other enjoys complete freedom. This makes absolutely no sense, and, in the end, amounts to rewarding one group for compliance with a behaviour that is of no medical value (in the model) – the value becomes purely political. So then, how blurred are the lines? How fast are they changing? Turning? Will the vaccinated suddenly get wiped off the travel roster? As shown in the next section, that reality is not so far fetched.

C. Baseline conditions are not fully developed nor adequately defined.

The authors do not explicitly state their baseline. From the tables presented and the papers referenced regarding initial assumptions, the initial conditions seem to be:

- Region: Ontario, Canada

- Proportion of population vaccinated: 80%

- Initial prevalence: 100 cases

- Timing: Post-Delta, with the Omicron variant emerging and just prior to an epidemic wave

- Factors such as season and population demographics do not seem to play a role in the model; no differentiation is made regarding type of vaccine administered.

D. The results follow from basic diffusion principles and are a simple projection of the authors' expectations

In the introduction of the paper, the authors state their central expectation regarding viral transmission:

> *Nonvaccination is expected to result in amplification of disease transmission in unvaccinated subpopulations, but the communicable nature of infectious diseases means that this also heightens risk for vaccinated populations, when vaccines confer imperfect immunity.*

The authors concocted a model that simply projects this expectation, as specified above, into a graphical representation. Nothing more.

E. Complete lack of diagnostic testing or benchmarking of results

The authors made no attempt to test the fit of their model to real-world data. Confidence intervals were not provided for the outputs (the deterministic model was not fit for this task). The authors provide no measures of reliability, validity, precision or confidence of the results. No statistical analysis was undertaken in the study.

Concern #3: Failure to capture real-world trends

While the authors failed to test their model, a quick visit to the Ontario Covid-19 website[10] provides an easy reality check.

As outlined in the previous section, the first wave of infections post-vaccination rollout, when almost 80% of the eligible population in Ontario was fully vaccinated (Dec 2021-Jan 2022), provides the most appropriate test-set to evaluate the model presented by Fisman et. al.

Figure 1 compares the incidence rates and incident cases that Ontario witnessed versus the simulated rates and cases produced by the Fisman et al. model under the intermediate like-with-like mixing scenario.

Across the range of all scenarios modeled, the simulated results indicated that (1) the risk of infection was markedly higher among the unvaccinated during the epidemic, as shown by disproportionately high incidence rates, and, (2) cases in the unvaccinated subpopulation accounted for a substantial proportion of infections during the epidemic wave.

As shown in the graphs below, not only are the simulated incident cases and rates off by orders of magnitude compared to those observed in the true epidemic wave,[11] the trends observed during the Dec/Jan epidemic were OPPOSITE to Fisman et al.'s simulated expectations.

Figure 1:[12] In Dec 2021-Jan 2022 the real-world version of Fisman et al.'s epidemic scenario played out.

A. Fisman et al. simulated (FAKE) scenario — COVID-19 Cases

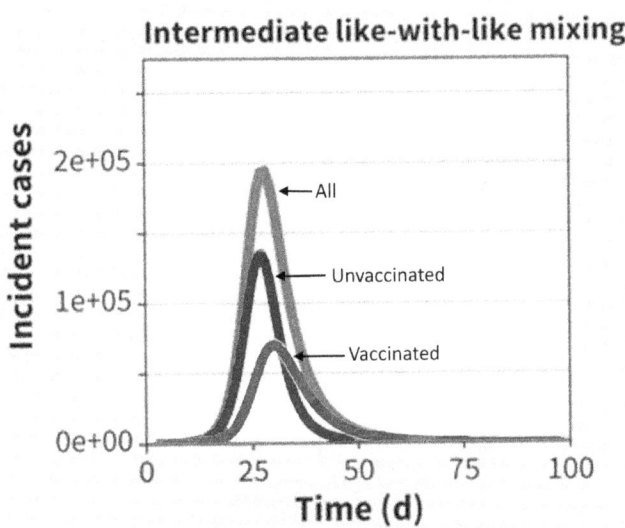

B. Ontario (REAL) data — COVID-19 Cases

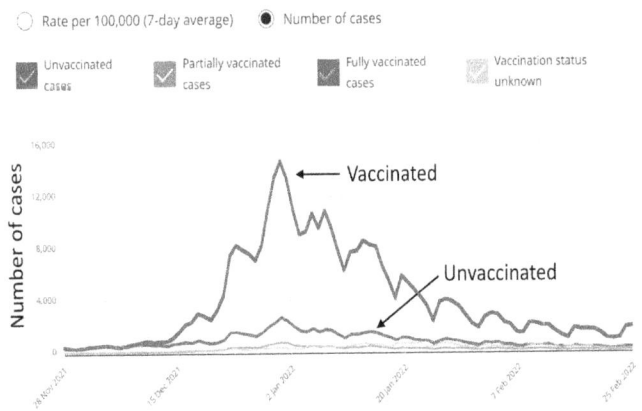

Figure 1 Continued:... Real-world observations were OPPOSITE to those simulated by Fisman et al.

C. Fisman et al. simulated (FAKE) scenario — COVID-19 Rates

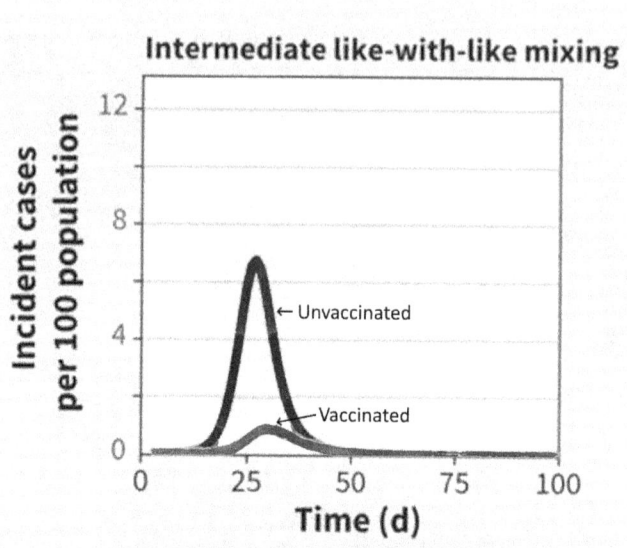

D. Ontario (REAL) data — COVID-19 Rates

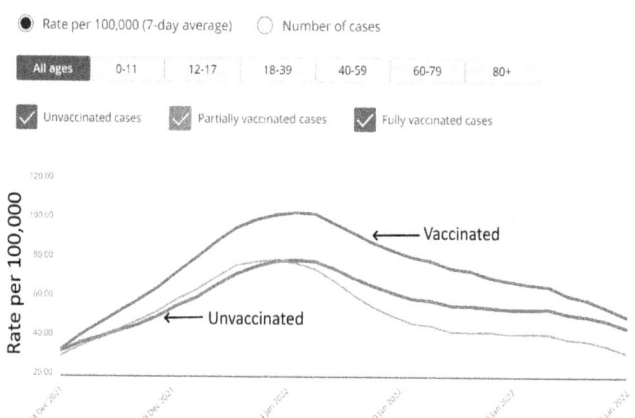

In reality, what we observed in the December 2021-January 2022 epidemic wave was the following (1) the incidence rates amongst the vaccinated population were disproportionately HIGHER than the unvaccinated and (2) cases in the vaccinated population account for the vast majority of Covid-19 infections. In short, Fisman et al.'s model failed completely. None of their scenarios captured the pattern observed in the true epidemic wave.

The trend of increased infection risk amongst the vaccinated population is not only being witnessed in Ontario, other countries have also reported this finding, including the UK. Even more worrisome are the current trends observed amongst the boosted population. Data from Ontario, UK and elsewhere indicate a susceptibility to infection that increases with each subsequent vaccine dose, with the boosted showing a marked increase as in Figure 2.[13] There are also concerns that any vaccine efficacy imparted from the vaccines begins to wane within increasingly shorter time frames. It is prudent for the scientific community to address this issue and openly discuss the implications of these striking, real-world observations.

Figure 2: Covid-19 Incidence rates by vaccine status

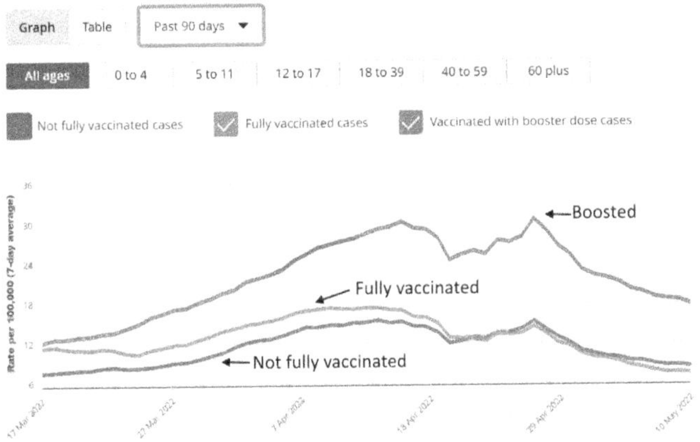

Ban the Boosted? Real data, pulled directly from the official Government of Ontario COVID-19 website, shows that incidence rates amongst persons who received their Covid booster shot far exceed those of the not fully vaccinated and double vaccinated. This trend has also been observed in other countries like the UK, casting doubt on the assertion that the booster vaccine enhances immunity and reduces onward transmission. Are they putting others at increased risk?

The emergence of the Omicron variant and the outbreak that ensued marked the first true test of Canada's vaccination efforts. The results were shocking: record levels of SARS-Cov-2 infections with greater incidence amongst the vaccinated.

The dissonance between what was expected and what transpired is so stunning that many refuse to acknowledge that it even happened. That certainly appears to be the case in the Fisman et al. study: no mention of the Dec/Jan epidemic, no attempt to create a model that simulates real-world transmission dynamics, and no attempt to test their "simple deterministic model."

Indeed, why bother with such basic scientific protocols if they are inconvenient?

The model was designed to simulate the outcomes that align with preconceived notions of how the virus and vaccines work. It provided a vehicle to influence public policy in a way that aligns with a political agenda. It passed the peer review process. It was published and passed on to major media outlets. And one week after publication, the study found its way into Canadian Parliament where Liberal MP, Adam van Koeverden, stood up and cited it as justification for travel restrictions against the unvaccinated.

This sequence of events is, of course, extremely dangerous. The harm that can come of such unscientific methods to influence policy cannot be overstated. The publication of Fisman et al.'s critically flawed population mixing model cannot be permitted to stand.

Concern #4: Misinterpretation of Results & Their Implications (Societal Harm)

The Fisman et al. study was **exploratory** in nature. The authors simplistic model projected their expectations of how a viral outbreak would play out under various population mixing scenarios *if* their understanding of transmission dynamics and vaccine efficacy were correct. It was not. A comparison of their projections with real-world data indicates that the authors' simplistic understanding is erroneous. Moreover, **any actions**

advocated by the authors based on their modelling are faulty and ill-advised.

The inability of Fisman et al. to recognize the failure of their model to adequately capture real-world transmission dynamics and viral incidence is consistent with the myopic approach they adopted – an approach that:

- Fails to consider the uncertainty in vaccine effectiveness, especially under emerging variants;

- Fails to consider the many risks and adverse consequences of vaccinating an entire population with new genetic vaccines that were developed, produced and administered at "remarkable speed" (as quoted in their mixing paper);

- Fails to consider the true limitations of their work;

- Fails to consider the potential for societal harm resulting from the adoption of their poorly constructed public policy suggestions;

- Fails to address the lack of evidence that strong government actions such as general lockdowns or the exclusion of unvaccinated individuals from restaurants, gyms, travel by plane or train etc. had any measurable benefit on covid transmission and incidence; and,

- Fails to discuss how heavy-handed measures compare to more moderate actions and treatments.

Given the influence of the authors in shaping public policy and advising on pandemic response,[14] these shortcomings are extremely concerning. What's more, the authors fail to acknowledge the disproportionate impacts of generalized pandemic measures on the young and healthy[15] as well as the immense harm that stems from measures that infringe on constitutional rights. These impacts affect both mental and physical well-being, individual finances and the greater economy, social cohesion and trust in government institutions. All these impacts need to be properly addressed, and that cannot be done with a simple mathematical model, a faulty one at that.

So where do we go from here?

By now, it should be clear that the underlying assumptions and modelling framework proposed by Fisman et al. have been proven false. **This finding, in itself, has tremendous value.**

Fisman et al. presented a model based on their understanding of SARS-CoV-2 transmission and vaccine efficacy. Indeed, the scenario they presented and their "findings" are consistent with the messaging and presumptions that have dominated our public health policies throughout the pandemic. This consistency with "accepted" expectations helps explain how the paper sailed through peer review, was published by CMAJ and why results were quickly disseminated to the public by corporate media. This demonstrates both the power and the danger of scientific bias and deeply rooted preconceived notions. It illustrates how glaring falsehoods and inconsistencies can escape the notice of established "experts" and it shows the willingness of media and politicians to uncritically accept "scientific" findings that suit their purpose.

This revelation signals that we need to stop for a moment, reflect on the pandemic strategy that has been adopted, and change course. We need to ask:

- Why are experts looking to simulated data for the answers when we already have the real data right in front of us?

- Why/how did Fisman et al. and so many other experts get things so wrong?

- What implication does this have on the "accepted" narrative regarding the vaccine program and vaccine effectiveness?

- If experts got this model and their findings so wrong when they literally had the real outcomes right in front of them, what else have they been wrong about?

- Don't the real-world observations from the Omicron wave demonstrate that federal vaccine mandates and travel restrictions against the unvaccinated are scientifically unsupported?

- Do the arguments supporting human rights violations that were presented in the Fisman et al. study justify greater restrictions be placed on vaccinated individuals, especially if boosted?

These are important questions and they should be addressed. Regarding the last two questions:

1. Yes, the real-world observations from the Omicron wave do, in fact, demonstrate **that federal vaccine mandates and travel restrictions** against the unvaccinated are scientifically **unsupported.**

2. The violation of fundamental human rights, whether for the unvaccinated subpopulation or vaccinated, should never be taken lightly. Indeed, there are safeguards written into the Constitution that are meant to protect the rights of citizens from government abuse and overreach. More on this in the section below.

We need to move forward in a more positive, comprehensive and beneficial manner. Objective, evidence-based science that **adheres to established protocols and ethics** is a powerful tool for understanding the world around us and can provide insight that benefits the health and safety of individuals and communities. It is important for universities and reputable journals to keep these principals at the forefront of their research efforts and peer-review processes to safeguard against unintended public harm and potential scientific fraud.

Concern #5: The danger of conflating reality with fiction

The assertions made in the interpretation section of the Fisman et al. paper moves the study from mere incompetence to the realm of scientific fraud and a vile attack on basic human rights.

Throughout the interpretation section of the Fisman et al. paper, the authors conflate reality with simulation and fact with fiction. Consider the following line taken from the interpretation section of the study

> "Many opponents of vaccine mandates have framed vaccine adoption as a matter of individual choice. However, we found that the *choices made by people* who forgo vaccination contribute

disproportionately to risk among those who do get vaccinated."

The authors did not show this. No people were involved in this study. No real-world observations were used at all. The statement points to a real-world issue, namely, freedom of individual choice. Then it claims that they found that *people* who forgo vaccination contribute disproportionately to risk. This flagrantly incriminating, unsubstantiated and fictitious "result" was quickly disseminated by the media.

The authors then continue along these faulty lines, making unwarranted assertions about population mixing and such, that ends on this "fact":

> The *fact* that this excess contribution to risk cannot be mitigated by high like-with-like mixing undermines the assertion that vaccine choice is best left to the individual and *supports strong public actions* aimed at enhancing vaccine uptake and limiting access to public spaces for unvaccinated people, because risk cannot be considered "self-regarding." There is ample precedent for public health regulation that protects the wider community from acquisition of communicable diseases, even if this protection comes at a cost of individual freedom."

A fact, a thing that is known or proved to be true:

Merriam-Webster

1(a): something that has actual existence; (b): an actual occurrence

2: a piece of information presented as having objective reality

3: the quality of being actual: ACTUALITY

Macmillan Dictionary

1: (COUNTABLE) a piece of true information

2: (UNCOUNTABLE) things that are true or that really happened, rather than things that are imaginary or not true

Other dictionaries such as the Cambridge Dictionary, Collins English Dictionary, Britannica Dictionary etc. all provide similar definitions.

What Fisman et al. present is not fact, it is fiction based on highly subjective, unscientific modelling that has no connection to reality whatsoever.

Not only is the "fact" statement presented by Fisman et al. deceiving and unjustified, it is highly irresponsible and potentially dangerous. The authors use the fictitious "fact" as a means to inadequately and inappropriately advise on public policy, advocating gross violations of human rights.

Contrary to claims made by Fisman et al., the study's findings <u>do not support</u> segregation, community exclusion of the unvaccinated or "strong public actions aimed at enhancing vaccine uptake." Such support is unwarranted and unethical. Moreover, the paper is an inappropriate forum to advocate public policy that undermines fundamental human rights, whimsically ignoring all the legal and ethical considerations built into the Canadian Constitution to protect such rights. How these fraudulent and unethical assertions escaped the peer-review process is unfathomable.

As mentioned in the above section, the Canadian Constitution was created to protect citizens from government abuse and overreach. While Section 1 of the Constitution includes a provision of reasonable limits to individual rights and freedoms when in the best interest of the greater community, any such limits must be demonstrably justified via the Oakes test. Indeed, the onus of proof is on the government and, to date, they have <u>failed to provide that proof</u>.

While a discussion regarding Oakes criteria and the lack of scientific evidence to support the federal vaccine mandate, travel restrictions and other covid measures is long overdue, it is beyond the scope of this critique. More pointedly, such constitutional considerations were also beyond the scope of the Fisman et. al study and any suggestion that a hypothetical, provably false simulation can justify the waving of constitutional rights and freedoms without such consideration is beyond absurd.

It is clear to me and many others that politicians have been misusing the name of "science" to justify circumventing the Constitution and their duty to provide the necessary evidence for the measures they impose. "Experts" have facilitated that abuse, most recently witnessed on Friday April 29th, 2022 when the Fisman et al. study made its way into parliamentary proceedings to support the federal travel restrictions against the unvaccinated.

This has to stop. The University of Toronto and CMAJ should not be party to it.

Science should not be used as a weapon to quash human rights and to circumvent the Constitution. Maintaining an objective scientific approach is vital when studying this pandemic and informing the public. Doing otherwise has tremendous potential to do harm and inadvertently increase misery and suffering.

Concern #6: The rampant spread of disinformation

A handful of model parameters in a spreadsheet hardly constitutes a person, yet many have conflated the entities of Fisman et al.'s simulation with real people. A fair question to ask is: Why is this so? News of the study spread rapidly to media outlets, who pushed articles such as the following to untold numbers of layman readers:

- *Merely hanging out with unvaccinated people puts the vaccinated at higher risk: study* by Eric Schank, *Salon (April 27, 2022)*

- *Unvaccinated people threaten the safety of individuals vaccinated against SARS-CoV-2* Reviewed by Emily Henderson, B.Sc., *News Medical (April 25, 2022)*

- *Unvaccinated People Increase Risk of Covid Infection Among Vaccinated, Study Finds* by Robert Hart, *Forbes (Apr 25, 2022)*

- *Unvaccinated disproportionately risk safety of those vaccinated against COVID-19, study shows* by Andrea Woo, *The Globe and Mail (April 25, 2022)*

Entities in Fisman et al.'s "unvaccinated" group are characterized mainly by a single parameter setting of 0.2 – the baseline immunity in unvaccinated people – which sets them apart from the "vaccinated" group. The Fisman et al. paper refers to this value as an assumption and is arbitrary. There is no artificial intelligence, social structure, or particularly complex interactions occurring between entities in this model. There is no real biology at play, or physics. There is no comparison with real situations or data. Every step is deterministic. These entities are completely "flat," abstract, and void of any connection to reality. Insight into exactly how they are conflated with real people can be gathered by a closer look at some of the articles:

- *Unvaccinated People Create Higher Risk for Vaccinated, Study Says* by Ralph Ellis, *WebMD (April 27, 2022)*

From the article:

"*People* who don't get vaccinated against COVID-19 are putting themselves in danger and also are creating a 'disproportionate' threat to the health of *vaccinated people*, even in places with high vaccination rates, says a study published in the Canadian Medical Association Journal."

- *Study: Unvaccinated People Increase COVID-19 Risk, Even Among Vaccinated People* by Roz Plater, *Healthline (April 25, 2022)*

From the article:

"Experts say COVID-19 risk increases when *unvaccinated people* mingle with vaccinated individuals."

"Dr. William Schaffner, a professor in the Division of Infectious Diseases at the Vanderbilt University School of Medicine in Tennessee said the study is a model, but the takeaways can be 'very, very instructive.'"

"We know that the virus can infect the vaccinated as well as unvaccinated people... but this model indicates, really with some clarity, *that unvaccinated people not only have obviously increased risk for themselves... but are more efficient transmitters... drivers or engines of transmission in the community,*" Schaffner told Healthline.

- *Mixing with the unvaccinated increases COVID-19 risk for the vaccinated, study finds* by Morgan Lowrie, *Canadian Press, Toronto Sun, Montreal Gazette, National Observer, Times Colonist (Apr 25, 2022)*

From the article:

"The research published Monday in the Canadian Medical Association Journal found that *vaccinated people* who mix with those who are not vaccinated have a significantly greater chance of being infected than those who *stick with people* who have received the shot."

These articles either contain quotes from the paper that make erroneous assertions about actual people that were never studied, and/or contain quotes from experts who have also confused Fisman et al.'s entities with people. That is, the public's misinterpretation is largely due to the erroneous manner in which the results were presented in the CMAJ paper, the erroneous connections to reality made or implied therein, and the dissemination pipeline. Moreover, the study – heavily centered on the Delta variant – was promoted as applicable to current day, despite the dominance of Omicron and despite the glaring contradiction of the model with Omicron infection case data. It is mindboggling how the authors could promote the hard-line views of this paper focused against the unvaccinated when current, readily available data indicates the much larger population of boosted individuals are showing multiple times (as much as three times[14]) the infection rate of unvaccinated individuals.

Clearly, the authors have generated a massive trail of misinformation, resulting in the propagation of fear, mistrust, and derisive attitudes towards a segment of the population in the real world who bear absolutely no resemblance to the entities in Fisman et al.'s model. The ethics of this endeavour must be addressed, and soon. Additionally, if some future version of this paper survives scrutiny and is not fully retracted, any references to actual people or reality should be removed from the paper. The first page should display a glaring warning that the results therein are highly oversimplified and do not relate to real events – past, present or projected.

Delving further into these and other articles that are based on the paper, it quickly becomes clear that the first author heavily promoted the work, leveraging the non-existing connections between the study and real people. For example,

- ***Unvaccinated people increase risk of COVID-19 infection among vaccinated: study*** by Irelyne Lavery, *Global News (April 25, 2022)*

Quote by David Fisman pulled from the article:

"We use models in a lot of different ways," said Fisman. "They're just simplified versions of *reality.*"

As noted in previous sections, Fisman et al.'s model cannot be considered as consistent with reality.

Another example appears in the article ***Merely hanging out with unvaccinated people puts the vaccinated at higher risk*** (as referenced above), speaking to the CMAJ article:

"I think it becomes reasonable to use vaccine mandates and passports as a measure that prevents the benefit of vaccines (in those who choose to be vaccinated) from being eroded by the choices of others," Fisman continued. "Striking a balance between the rights of individuals and rights of communities is pretty much bread-and-butter public health, so it's unclear to me why this would be contentious. There is no fundamental right to spread tuberculosis, typhoid or syphilis, for example."

In the above quote, Fisman likens normally-healthy unvaccinated people to carriers of tuberculosis, typhoid, and syphilis. Perhaps Dr. Fisman can clarify how the SARS-Cov-2 population mixing study is related to syphilis transmission and vaccination. Is there even a syphilis vaccine available? Is a study regarding the transmission of syphilis forthcoming that will shed light on this link?

These appear to be more false comparisons, the goal of which is to cast individuals labelled as unvaccinated in poor light. Comments of this nature to media outlets expose intent, and elevate the disseminated material from misinformation to disinformation.

In short, the ramifications of the Fisman et al. publication, just days off the press, have been immensely harmful and have caused an even greater rift in in an already divided society. Media, politicians and the public have confused the fiction presented by Fisman et al., and published by CMAJ, as fact.

Not surprisingly, the prevailing takeaways from the study are that unvaccinated people threaten the safety of the vaccinated, they are "drivers" of disease,[16] and that it's best to "stick to your own kind." The misleading headlines noted above represent a mere sample of the disinformation that is running rampant.

An immediate remedy must be sought to end the disinformation and put a stop to further harm accruing from this study.

Concern #7: Blatant scientific and research misconduct

As outlined in the University of Toronto's Policy on Ethical Conduct in Research, the university expects all faculty, students and those holding a university post to adhere to the highest standards of ethical conduct in every aspect of research. Moreover, the university policy complies with the requirements of the Tri-Agencies (CIHR, NSERC or SSHRC) whose framework promotes scholarly and scientific rigour as well as honesty and accountability in the dissemination of knowledge.

Allegations specific to the University's Framework to Address Allegations of Research Misconduct include:

A. Fraud including the fabrication and falsification of data and results - two of the most severe violations of research integrity.

Data fabrication is the act of making up data and reporting the made-up data as a true reflection of events. This often occurs when a researcher fills out the experiment with personal assumed data (Kang and Hwang, 2020). An example of fabrication includes artificially creating data when it should be collected from an actual experiment or observation (Northern

Illinois University, 2022). The fabrication of data is a particularly blatant form of misconduct; it is a deliberate attempt to deceive others (Online Ethics Center, 2022).

Falsification involves a deliberate manipulation the research process to produce a desired result, including leaving out data that goes against a desired result (Kuali,2021).

Falsification and fabrication are dangerous to the public as they can result in people giving and receiving incorrect medical advice; relying on falsified data can lead to death or injury or lead patients to take a drug, treatment, or use a medical device that is less effective than perceived (Poutoglidou et al. 2022).

> *Fisman et al. concocted a simulation to produce outcomes that align with their personal beliefs, they omitted any reference to readily available real-world data that completely contradicts their results, then proceeded to state the fabricated results as fact. Furthermore, they advocated for human rights violations to be put into public policy based on their fictitious findings.*

B. Willfully misrepresenting and misinterpreting findings resulting from conducting research activities.

As mentioned in previous sections, the authors make numerous misrepresentations and misinterpretations of findings. Moreover, the following indicate that the misrepresentations are willful:

i. The authors show overt bias and make inappropriate disparaging comments indicating personal prejudice.

ii. Within one week of the publication, over a dozen rebukes submitted by 22 researchers and health care professionals were brought to the attention of the authors and posted on the CMAJ website. These serious concerns have gone largely dismissed. On May 3rd, 2022 the authors acknowledged that they had received criticism regarding their incorrect interpretation of model results, their incorrect choice of parameters and that their model is stoking hatred against those who choose to remain unvaccinated against SARS-CoV-2. Instead of heeding these warnings and giving these concerns their due diligence, the authors suggest that any errors lie with the (mis)interpretation or lack of modelling competency of those critiquing the paper. Moreover, despite several medical doctors and researchers pointing out the inconsistency of the study's findings with real-world data, the authors double-down on their erroneous findings (CMAJ, 2022).

iii. The main author has, on several occasions and through various media outlets, stated the findings as fact or a reflection of reality knowing that wasn't the case.

iv. The authors list mathematical modelling as a key area of expertise; the main author is a tenured professor who teaches mathematical epidemiology. Certainly, such individuals would understand rudimentary model building, interpretation of results and inference.

v. The authors list several substantive conflicts of interest that align with the fabricated results.

The use of this critically flawed work and fraudulent claims to target and penalize a segment of society is not only harmful to the group it seeks to punish, but to society as a whole. By reinforcing a false premise regarding transmission and infection, it hinders actual progress from being made and that affects the health and wellbeing of everyone.

C. Lack of sufficient scientific rigour.

The main author, Dr. David Fisman, is a tenured professor of epidemiology who highlights mathematical modelling & simulation along with decision analysis & cost-effectiveness analysis as research interests. A co-author, Dr. Ashleigh Tuite, is an infectious disease epidemiologist and mathematical modeler. In particular, she is interested in the use of mathematical models to synthesize and communicate complex information and uncertainty.

It is difficult to reconcile the alleged expertise of the authors with such a poorly constructed study that fails to adhere to the most basic research protocols. This does not bode well for the reputation of the University of Toronto and it undermines the field of mathematical epidemiology.

Recall that it was the mortality projections based on Professor Neil Ferguson's seriously flawed epidemiological model that sparked global lockdowns in 2020, including here in Canada. These lockdowns have had a detrimental impact on our health and well-being as well as the economy. The massive influence of the projections that came from this one study — projections that were overstated by orders of magnitude — was largely a result of who reported them. As Mark Landler and Stephen Castle wrote in the New York Times: "It wasn't so much the numbers themselves, frightening though they were, as who reported them: Imperial College London." The Times articled noted that, with the professor's ties to the WHO, Imperial was "treated as a sort of gold standard, its mathematical models feeding directly into government policies." (Landler and Castle, 2020; St. Onge and Campan, 2020).

Ferguson's report, based on a clearly faulty model, advocated for radical lockdowns and strict social distancing until a vaccine was available. Now Fisman et al.'s fraudulent report, written by faculty members out of University of Toronto and published by CMAJ, vilifies and advocates for human rights violations against individuals that, in reality, have shown and continue to show (as of this writing) reduced infection rates compared to the vaccinated (especially those who received a booster shot).

The harm that comes from such scientific misconduct is massive, especially during a global pandemic where scientific results can quickly be incorporated into government policy that affects tens of millions of lives.

The authors' credibility is clearly compromised in this area and this brings into question any previous work, recommendations, and advocacy these authors have done regarding the pandemic. All such work should be reviewed for errors and bias, especially in regards to Covid-19 vaccination or anything derived from mathematical modelling exercises done in part, wholly, or influenced by any of the three authors.

Bottom Line: A RETRACTION and INVESTIGATION are in order

The assertion made by the authors of Fisman et al. that the unvaccinated contribute disproportionately to risk among those who do get vaccinated is completely unfounded. It is direct result of a fabricated model that flips reality. Indeed, the data posted on the official Ontario Covid website shows that during the Omicron surge in Dec 2021 – Jan 2022, the incidence rate was disproportionately greater amongst the vaccinated group. Not only has this trend continued, individuals who've received the booster dose show even greater risk of infection.

> **The Fisman et al. study concocted a model simulation that FLIPPED reality, then proceeded to inform policy based on this inverted, false reality. More specifically, the study leveraged a false premise to support public policy aimed at enhancing vaccine uptake and limiting access to public spaces for unvaccinated people.**

This study must be retracted, immediately, and denounced by both the University of Toronto and CMAJ. As competent, ethical scientists, we cannot pretend that the epidemic wave in Dec/Jan never happened and simply overwrite it with a fake simulation that says the opposite.

Moreover, I am calling on the University of Toronto to investigate David N. Fisman, Afia Amoako and Ashleigh R. Tuite for research misconduct. The affiliations of the main author with the Ontario Science Table, Pfizer and other pharma companies, along with the affiliation of Tuite with the Centre for Immunization Readiness (Public Health Agency of Canada) and the affiliation of all authors with the Dalla Lana School of Public Health (University of Toronto) call into question the prevailing advice our public health officials have been given, the intent behind that advice and the consequences of "expert" incompetence or deception.

Notes

---

[1] The research was supported by a grant to David Fisman; 2019 COVID-19 rapid researching funding OV4-170360

[2] David N. Fisman, Afia Amoako, Ashleigh R. Tuite. Impact of population mixing between vaccinated and unvaccinated subpopulations on infectious disease dynamics: implications for SARS-CoV-2 transmission. CMAJ 2022;194:E573-E580

[3] The date has been corrected to April 29th, 2022. The date appearing in the original copies sent to the institutions was May 2nd, 2022.

[4] The Competing Interests section of the paper notes, "David Fisman has served as a volunteer scientist on the Ontario COVID-19 Science Advisory Table and has served as a legal expert on issues related to COVID-19 epidemiology for the Elementary Teachers Federation of Ontario and the Registered Nurses Association of Ontario. He has also served on advisory boards related to influenza and SARS-CoV-2 vaccines for Seqirus, Pfizer, AstraZeneca and Sanofi-Pasteur Vaccines. Ashleigh Tuite was employed by the Public Health Agency of Canada when the research was conducted."

[5] Within one week of publication, rebukes by 22 other researchers and health care professionals had already been submitted and posted on the Canadian Medical Association Journal website; https://www.cmaj.ca/content/194/16/E573/tab-e-letters.

[6] Fisman et al. make the statement without: (i) providing any evidence or discussion as to whether the cancellation of elective surgeries was necessary or

warranted; (ii) presenting any evidence supporting disproportionate hospitalization or increased health care service amongst the unvaccinated, and (iii) without consideration of <u>all-cause</u> hospitalizations and <u>all-cause</u> mortality. It should be noted that since vaccine outcomes have not been actively tracked and monitored, one <u>cannot establish a net reduction</u> in hospitalization or death due to vaccination.

[7] The value 0.8 used for vaccine effectiveness does not appear to follow directly from the sources referenced by Fisman et al. I could not find an actual reference to the 0.4 value used for Omicron.

From the preprint Effectiveness of COVID-19 vaccines against Omicron or Delta infection (2021.12.30.21268565v1.full): "... receipt of 2 doses of COVID-19 vaccines was not protective against Omicron infection at any point in time, and VE was −38% (95%CI, −61%, −18%) 120-179 days and −42% (95%CI, −69%, −19%) 180-239 days after the second dose. VE against Omicron was 37% (95%CI, 19-50%) ≥7 days after receiving an mRNA vaccine for the third dose. Findings were consistent for any combination of 2 mRNA vaccines and 2 doses of BNT162b2 for the primary series (Table S1, Figure S1)."

[8] There appears to be no basis for the 0.2 estimate used as the base reference for natural immunity amongst the unvaccinated.

[9] Once again, Fisman et al. fails to acknowledge possible harms. It should be noted that adverse vaccine reactions are not being actively tracked; causal relationships between injury and covid vaccination have been established; and, we do not know the extent of long-term adverse effects. Vaccine benefits need to be properly weighed against such unintended harms.

[10] For the Ontario Covid-19 data: unvaccinated is defined as the number of cases where: people did not have any vaccine dose, or where symptoms started between 0 and less than 14 days after receiving the first dose of a COVID-19 vaccine; Partially vaccinated cases is defined as the number of cases where symptoms started: 14 days or more after receiving the first dose of a 2-dose vaccine series, or between 0 and less than 14 days after receiving the second dose of a 2-dose vaccine series; Fully vaccinated cases is defined as the number of cases where symptoms started 14 days or more after receiving: the second dose of a 2-dose vaccine series, or a single-dose vaccine series (for example, Janssen).

[11] It should be noted that actual infection rates can be quite different than reported case rates, as was the situation early in the pandemic. However, with increased testing, the two quantities tend to converge (this is why we have seen a convergence of Case Fatality Rate with Infection Fatality Rate). Note that the authors speak to cases but they may be referring to actual infections; it is unclear. This conflating of terminology is rampant throughout the paper.

Another example of conflation is in regards to vaccine effectiveness versus efficacy versus immunity. These terms have separate meanings yet seem to be used interchangeably within the paper

[12] REF: Simulated plots appear as Figures 1C & 1D in Fisman et al. (2022). Plots depicting Ontario incident rates and cases by vaccination status were screenshots taken from https://covid-19.ontario.ca/data, retrieved in January 2022 and May 2022 (via the waybackmachine), respectively.

[13] Not fully vaccinated cases: Number of cases where: people did not have any vaccine dose; symptoms started after receiving the first dose of a 2-dose COVID-19 vaccine; symptoms started between 0 and less than 14 days after receiving the first dose of a single-dose vaccine series (for example, Janssen); symptoms started between 0 and less than 14 days after receiving the second dose of a 2-dose vaccine series. Fully vaccinated cases: Number of cases where symptoms started 14 days or more after receiving: the second dose of a 2-dose vaccine series, or a single-dose vaccine series (for example, Janssen). Vaccinated-with booster dose cases: Fully vaccinated people with one or more booster dose administered at least 14 days before symptoms started

[14] The Competing Interests section of the paper notes, "David Fisman has served as a volunteer scientist on the Ontario COVID-19 Science Advisory Table and has served as a legal expert on issues related to COVID-19 epidemiology for the Elementary Teachers Federation of Ontario and the Registered Nurses Association of Ontario. He has also served on advisory boards related to influenza and SARS-CoV-2 vaccines for Seqirus, Pfizer, AstraZeneca and Sanofi-Pasteur Vaccines. Ashleigh Tuite was employed by the Public Health Agency of Canada when the research was conducted."

[15] The risk profile of covid-19 increases by several orders of magnitude from the youngest in the community to the eldest. Conversely, in the context of long-term safety, the risk profile of the vaccine is largest for younger age groups and lowest for the elderly. Other factors such as underlying health, gender, occupation and work environment also impact these risk profiles. Pandemic measures and vaccine mandates that completely ignore these factors and are applied in a blanket manner cannot be seen as minimal. When risk changes by orders of magnitude between identifiable groups, strategic measures and strategic allocation of resources will yield optimal benefit while a blanket approach results in disproportionate impacts across groups and is both wasteful and potentially disastrous. This follows from basic principals of mathematics and optimization.

For most individuals, SARS-CoV-2 poses little risk of serious disease and it has been likened to the common cold. The risk of severe disease is, however, a concern for a small and identifiable subpopulation, namely the elderly and those with underlying health issues.

Note that the infection fatality rate (IFR) is estimated to be in the ballpark of 0.05% for those under 70 years old (Ioannidis JPA. Infection fatality rate of COVID-19 inferred from seroprevalence data. Bull World Health Organ. 2020 Oct 14 [Epub ahead of print]).

CDC best estimate of IFR (Infection fatality ratio) in the US as of Sept. 10, 2020: Age 0-19 years: 0.00003; Age 20-49 years; Age 0.0002; Age 50-69 years: 0.005; Age 70+ years: 0.054. Updated IFR estimates as of Mar. 19, 2021: Age 0-17: 0.00002; Age 18-49: 0.0005; Age 50-64: 0.006; Age 65+: 0.09 (COVID-19 Pandemic Planning Scenarios: CDC).

[16] Once again, real-world data indicate the opposite may be the case, see COVID-19 Alberta Statistics, (retrieved via The Wayback Machine - https://web.archive.org/web/20220110084941/https://www.alberta.ca/stats/covid-19-alberta-statistics.htm).

There is evidence of increased susceptibility to SARS-CoV-2 within the 14 days of an individual's first inoculation. This suggests that vaccination may drive transmission, especially in the absence of policy or vaccination protocols that warn individuals of this increased risk or that do not attempt to limit exposure to the virus during this time. This also demonstrates potential bias in labeling those who experience covid symptoms within 14 days of their first or second inoculation as "unvaccinated" as is the case for the data presented on the official Ontario Cov-19 website.

Another indication that vaccination may help drive infection appeared early during the Pfizer clinical trials. See: Vaccines and Related Biological Products Advisory Committee Meeting December 10, 2020 FDA Briefing Document Pfizer-BioNTech COVID-19 Vaccine: "Clinical laboratory tests (hematology, chemistries) were assessed in study BNT162-01 and C4591001 phase 1. The only common laboratory abnormality reported throughout the studies was transient decreases in lymphocytes 1-3 days after Dose 1, which increased in frequency with increasing dose, were mostly Grade 1-2, generally normalized at the next laboratory assessment 6-8 days after Dose 1." Also within the report: "Suspected COVID-19 cases that occurred within 7 days after any vaccination were 409 in the vaccine group vs. 287 in the placebo group."

References

CDC. "COVID-19 Pandemic Planning Scenarios." Sept. 10, 2020; Revised March 19, 2021. https://www.cdc.gov/coronavirus/2019-ncov/hcp/planning-scenarios.html.

Chemaitelly, Hiam, Patrick Tang, Mohammad R. Hasan et al. "Waning of BNT162b2 Vaccine Protection against SARS-CoV-2 Infection in Qatar." N Engl J Med 2021; 385:e83. December 9, 2021. DOI: 10.1056/NEJMoa2114114.

CMAJ. "Responses (Re: Impact of population mixing between vaccinated and unvaccinated subpopulations on infectious disease dynamics: implications for SARS-CoV-2 transmission)." Accessed May 16, 2022. https://www.cmaj.ca/content/194/16/E573/tab-e-letters#re-impact-of-population-mixing-between-vaccinated-and-unvaccinated-subpopulations-on-infectious-disease-dynamics-implications-for-sars-cov-2-transmission.

Collier, Roger. "Scientific misconduct or criminal offence ?" *CMAJ*. November 17, 2015 187 (17) 1273-1274. https://doi.org/10.1503/cmaj.109-5171.

Crichton, Michael. "Aliens Cause Global Warming." Caltech Michelin Lecture. January 17, 2003. https://stephenschneider.stanford.edu/Publications/PDF_Papers/Crichton2003.pdf.

Ellis, Ralph. "Unvaccinated People Create Higher Risk for Vaccinated,

Study Says." *WebMD*. April 27, 2022. https://www.webmd.com/vaccines/covid-19-vaccine/news/20220427/unvaccinated-people-create-higher-risk-for-vaccinated-study-says.

Fisman, David N., Afia Amoako, and Ashleigh R. Tuite. "Impact of population mixing between vaccinated and unvaccinated subpopulations on infectious disease dynamics: implications for SARS-CoV-2 transmission." *CMAJ*. April 25, 2022 194 (16) E573-E580. DOI: https://doi.org/10.1503/cmaj.212105.

Government of Canada. "Health Canada Decision-Making Framework for Identifying, Assessing, and Managing Health Risks - August 1, 2000." Accessed on January 22, 2023. https://www.canada.ca/en/health-canada/corporate/about-health-canada/reports-publications/health-products-food-branch/health-canada-decision-making-framework-identifying-assessing-managing-health-risks.html#a35.

Government of Canada. "Immunization Partnership Fund - Canada.ca." November 15, 2022. https://www.canada.ca/en/public-health/services/immunization-vaccine-priorities/immunization-partnership-fund.html#wb-auto-4.

Hart, Robert. "Unvaccinated People Increase Risk of Covid Infection Among Vaccinated, Study Finds." *Forbes*. April 25, 2022. https://www.forbes.com/sites/roberthart/2022/04/25/unvaccinated-people-increase-risk-of-covid-infection-among-vaccinated-study-finds/?sh=3a0da7a124a3.

Henderson, Emily. "Unvaccinated people threaten the safety of individuals vaccinated against SARS-CoV-2." *News Medical*. April 25, 2022. https://www.news-medical.net/news/20220425/Unvaccinated-people-threaten-the-safety-of-individuals-vaccinated-against-SARS-CoV-2.aspx.

Kalvapalle, Rahul. "U of T partners with Moderna to advance research in RNA science and technology." University of Toronto News. April 7, 2022. https://www.utoronto.ca/news/u-t-partners-moderna-advance-research-rna-science-and-technology.

Kang, Eungoo and Hee-Joong Hwang. "The Consequences of Data Fabrication and Falsification among Researchers." *Journal of Research and Publication Ethics* Vol 1 No 2 (September 05, 2020), 7-10, JEL Classification Code : I29, O30, O39. https://www.koreascience.or.kr/article/JAKO202027265688897.pdf.

Kuali. "Research Misconduct: Why We Need to Take it Seriously." Kuali Higher Ed Software - Higher Ed SaaS Solutions. October 20, 2021. https://www.kuali.co/post/research-misconduct-why-we-need-to-take-it-seriously.

Landler, Mark and Stephen Castle. "Behind the Virus Report That Jarred the U.S. and the U.K. to Action." *The New York Times*. March 17, 2020. https://www.nytimes.com/2020/03/17/world/europe/coronavirus-imperial-college-johnson.html.

Lavery, Irelyne. "Unvaccinated people increase risk of COVID-19 infection among vaccinated: study." *Global News*. April 25, 2022. https://globalnews.ca/news/8783380/unvaccinated-vaccinated-covid-risk-canadian-study/.

Lowrie, Morgan. "Mixing with the unvaccinated increases COVID-19 risk for the vaccinated, study finds." *Montreal Gazette*. April 25, 2022. https://montrealgazette.com/pmn/news-pmn/canada-news-pmn/mixing-with-unvaccinated-increases-covid-19-risk-for-vaccinated-people-study-finds-2/wcm/964efac0-7226-46c2-b546-2e4c57d7e036.

Lowrie, Morgan. "Mixing with the unvaccinated increases COVID-19 risk for the vaccinated, study finds." *National Observer*. April 25, 2022. https://www.nationalobserver.com/2022/04/25/news/mixing-unvaccinated-risk-covid-vaccinated.

Lowrie, Morgan. "Mixing with the unvaccinated increases COVID-19 risk for the vaccinated, study finds." *Times Colonist*. April 25, 2022. https://www.timescolonist.com/national-news/mixing-with-unvaccinated-increases-covid-19-risk-for-vaccinated-people-study-finds-5295746.

Lowrie, Morgan. "Mixing with the unvaccinated increases COVID-19 risk for the vaccinated, study finds." *Toronto Sun.* April 25, 2022. https://torontosun.com/health/mixing-with-the-unvaccinated-increases-covid-19-risk-for-the-vaccinated-study-finds.

Majdoubi, Abdelilah, Christina Michalski, Sarah E. O'Connell et al. "A majority of uninfected adults show preexisting antibody reactivity against SARS-CoV-2." *JCI insight.* March 15, 2021. https://insight.jci.org/articles/view/146316.

Mencken, H.L. "A Mencken Chrestomathy." Knopf. New York, 1962. First published January 1, 1949.

Northern Illinois University. "Fabrication or Falsification: Academic Integrity Tutorial for Students." Accessed on May 20, 2022. https://www.niu.edu/academic-integrity/students/cheating/fabrication-or-falsification.shtml.

Online Ethics Center. "Overly Ambitious Researchers - Fabricating Data." Accessed on May 20, 2022. https://onlineethics.org/cases/ethics-science-classroom/overly-ambitious-researchers-fabricating-data.

Panel on Responsible Conduct of Research. "Tri-Agency Framework: Responsible Conduct of Research (2016)." Government of Canada. Accessed on January 24, 2023. https://rcr.ethics.gc.ca/eng/framework-cadre.html#a2-1.

Plater, Roz. "Study: Unvaccinated People Increase COVID-19 Risk, Even Among Vaccinated People." *Healthline.* April 25, 2022. https://www.healthline.com/health-news/study-unvaccinated-people-increase-covid-19-risk-even-among-vaccinated-people.

Poutoglidou, Frideriki, Marios Stavrakas, Nikolaos Tsetsos, Alexandros Poutoglidis, Aikaterini Tsentemeidou, Georgios Fyrmpas, Petros D. Karkos. "Fraud and Deceit in Medical Research: Insights and Current Perspectives." *Voices in Bioethics.* Jan 26, 2022. DOI https://doi.org/10.52214/

vib.v8i.8940.

Schank, Eric. "Merely hanging out with unvaccinated people puts the vaccinated at higher risk: study." *Salon.* April 27, 2022. https://www.salon.com/2022/04/27/unvaccinated-risk/.

St. Onge, Peter and Gaël Campan. "The Flawed COVID-19 Model That Locked Down Canada." Montreal Economic Institute. June 4, 2020. https://www.iedm.org/the-flawed-covid-19-model-that-locked-down-canada/.

UK Health Security Agency. "COVID-19 vaccine surveillance report Week 11." Publishing.service.gov.uk. March 17, 2022. https://assets.publishing.service.gov.uk/government/uploads/system/uploads/attachment_data/file/1061532/Vaccine_surveillance_report_-_week_11.pdf.

University of Toronto Dalla Lana School of Public Health Faculty Database. "Fisman, David N." December 2, 2020. https://www.dlsph.utoronto.ca/faculty-profile/fisman-david-n/.

University of Toronto Dalla Lana School of Public Health Faculty Database. "Tuite, Ashleigh." December 4, 2020. https://www.dlsph.utoronto.ca/faculty-profile/tuite-ashleigh/.

University of Toronto. "Submit a Research Integrity Complaint." Accessed on January 24, 2023. https://research.utoronto.ca/research-integrity/submit-research-integrity-complaint.

Woo, Andrea. "Unvaccinated disproportionately risk safety of those vaccinated against COVID-19, study shows." *The Globe and Mail.* April 25, 2022. https://www.theglobeandmail.com/canada/article-unvaccinated-covid-risk-for-vaccinated-canada/.

About the Author

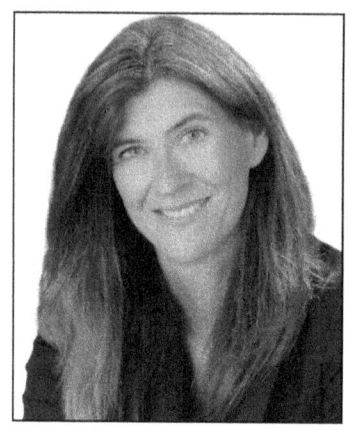

Regina holds a PhD in Statistics from the University of Western Ontario with a strong background in the sciences. She has served as a consultant to medical practitioners, social scientists and various levels of government. She also served as the principal statistician for an Ottawa-based economics consulting firm that specialized in econometrics, program evaluation, business case development and risk-benefit-options analysis.

As project manager and lead analyst, Dr. Watteel routinely engaged with stakeholder groups to deliver comprehensive solutions from early needs assessments and metrics development through to data collection, performance measurement, statistical analysis and the dissemination of findings, including implications and limitations. She has taught both undergraduate and graduate level university courses in multivariate statistical analysis, data analysis and engineering statistics.

Dr. Watteel's career path took a dramatic turn following a motor vehicle accident in which a substance impaired driver plowed into her while she was putting groceries in the trunk of her vehicle. Ultimately, Dr. Watteel stepped down from her position to focus on rehabilitation, health and her three children. She also took the opportunity to branch out and pursue aspirations in the publishing business. During the pandemic, concerns over the censorship of important scientific information and a government course of action that seemed to be moving in a direction of maximal harm and risk prompted a passionate return as a statistical sleuth.

Since March 2020, Regina N. Watteel has monitored the evolving world-wide pandemic data, government responses and emerging scientific findings. Early on, it became apparent to Dr. Watteel that the government's actions were not based on sound decision-making practices and were at odds with their own risk management framework, which they appeared to have abandoned completely. She has been outspoken about the need for transparency and the importance of adhering to a rational, evidence-based approach that is open to scrutiny.

Printed in the USA
CPSIA information can be obtained
at www.ICGtesting.com
LVHW040348310124
770470LV00004B/51